EPI DIET FOOD LIST FOR BEGINNERS

Revitalize Your Nutrition: A Culinary Journey to Wellness

Kerry Motter

Copyright © 2024

All Rights Are Reserved

The content in this book may not be reproduced, duplicated, or transferred without the express written permission of the author or publisher. Under no circumstances will the publisher or author be held liable or legally responsible for any losses, expenditures, or damages incurred directly or indirectly as a consequence of the information included in this book.

Legal Remarks

Copyright protection applies to this publication. It is only intended for personal use. No piece of this work may be modified, distributed, sold, quoted, or paraphrased without the author's or publisher's consent.

Disclaimer Statement

Please keep in mind that the contents of this booklet are meant for educational and recreational purposes. Every effort has been made to offer accurate, up-to-date, reliable, and thorough information. There are, however, no stated or implied assurances of any kind. Readers understand that the author is providing competent counsel. The content in this book originates from several sources. Please seek the opinion of a competent professional before using any of the tactics outlined in this book. By reading this book, the reader agrees that the author will not be held accountable for any direct or indirect damages resulting from the use of the information contained therein, including, but not limited to, errors, omissions, or inaccuracies.

Table of Contents

INTRODUCTION 1

UNDERSTANDING THE EPI DIET 3

    What is EPI? 3

    Importance of Diet in EPI Management 4

    Goals of the EPI Diet 5

FUNDAMENTALS OF THE EPI DIET 7

    Overview of the EPI Diet 7

    Key Principles and Guidelines 7

    Foods to Include and Avoid 9

    Importance of Nutrient Absorption 10

GETTING STARTED WITH THE EPI DIET 12

    Planning Your Meals 12

    Shopping Tips for EPI-Friendly Foods 13

    Meal Prep and Cooking Techniques 14

EPI DIET FOOD GROUPS 16

    Lean Meats 16

    Poultry 16

    Fish and Seafood 17

    Plant-Based Protein Sources 17

    Healthy Fats and Oils 18

Essential Fatty Acids..18

Cooking Oils and Fats to Choose..18

Carbohydrates and Fiber 19

Whole Grains 19

Fruits and Vegetables..19

Legumes and Beans 20

TIPS FOR SUCCESS AND ADDITIONAL RESOURCES 21

Tips for Adhering to the EPI Diet...21

Eating Out and Social Situations 22

Managing Digestive Symptoms 23

Staying Motivated and Consistent 24

Additional Resources and Support..24

BREAKFAST RECIPES 26

Savory Breakfast Quinoa Bowl 26

Blueberry Almond Chia Pudding..27

Spinach and Feta Omelette 28

Avocado Toast with Smoked Salmon.....................................29

Greek Yogurt Parfait with Berries and Granola 30

Egg and Vegetable Breakfast Burrito 31

Quinoa Breakfast Porridge..32

Sweet Potato and Black Bean Breakfast Hash........................33

Coconut Chia Seed Pudding 35

Quinoa Breakfast Bowl 36

Smoked Salmon and Avocado Toast 37

Greek Yogurt Parfait 38

Spinach and Feta Omelette 39

Blueberry Almond Chia Pudding 40

Spinach and Mushroom Breakfast Frittata 41

Overnight Oats with Berries and Almonds 42

Turkey and Vegetable Breakfast Hash 44

Green Breakfast Smoothie Bowl 45

Avocado and Tomato Breakfast Toast 46

SNACKS RECIPES 48

Chia Seed Pudding 48

Apple and Peanut Butter Slices 49

Greek Yogurt with Berries and Honey 49

Vegetable Sticks with Hummus 50

Trail Mix 51

Energy Balls 52

Vegetable Sushi Rolls 53

Roasted Chickpeas 55

Caprese Skewers 56

Hummus Stuffed Bell Peppers...57

Quinoa Salad with Avocado and Chickpeas.................................58

Turkey and Cheese Roll-Ups..59

Greek Yogurt Parfait..60

Zucchini and Carrot Fritters...61

Edamame and Avocado Dip 62

Hummus and Veggie Wraps...63

Banana and Almond Butter Bites 64

Greek Yogurt with Honey and Walnuts...65

Cottage Cheese with Pineapple...66

Roasted Edamame..66

DESSERTS RECIPES 68

Fruit Salad with Honey-Lime Dressing 68

Dark Chocolate Avocado Mousse 69

Baked Apples with Cinnamon 70

Chia Seed Pudding...71

Baked Banana Oatmeal Cups...72

Blueberry Oatmeal Cookies..73

Chia Seed Chocolate Pudding..75

Baked Peach Crisp 76

Coconut Yogurt Parfait..77

Frozen Banana Bites 78

Berry Chia Seed Pudding 79

Cinnamon Baked Apples.. 80

Coconut Almond Date Balls 82

Greek Yogurt with Honey and Pistachios 83

Baked Pears with Cinnamon and Walnuts 83

Almond Butter Banana Bites 85

Greek Yogurt Parfait with Berries 86

Chocolate Avocado Pudding... 87

Fruit Salad with Mint Honey Dressing 88

Baked Cinnamon Apple Slices 89

SEAFOOD RECIPES 91

Grilled Lemon Herb Salmon... 91

Baked Lemon Garlic Shrimp 92

Pan-Seared Scallops with Lemon Butter Sauce 93

Grilled Garlic Herb Shrimp Skewers 94

Baked Lemon Dijon Salmon... 96

Lemon Garlic Shrimp Pasta 97

Grilled Salmon with Avocado Salsa 98

Shrimp and Vegetable Stir-Fry 99

Tuna Salad Stuffed Avocados 101

Baked Cod with Lemon Herb Crust...102

Herb-Crusted Baked Salmon 103

Coconut Shrimp with Mango Salsa 104

Tilapia Piccata...106

Grilled Halibut with Lemon Herb Sauce 107

Lemon Garlic Shrimp with Quinoa..108

Baked Cod with Tomato Basil Relish...109

Cajun Grilled Shrimp Skewers 111

Salmon Cakes with Avocado Yogurt Sauce 112

SOUP RECIPES 114

Creamy Butternut Squash Soup...114

Lentil and Vegetable Soup...115

Coconut Curry Shrimp Soup..116

Tomato Basil Soup...118

Miso Soup with Tofu and Seaweed 119

Creamy Spinach and Chickpea Soup 120

Vegetable Quinoa Soup 122

Ginger Carrot Soup..123

Creamy Mushroom Soup 124

Lentil Vegetable Soup..126

Detox Lentil Soup..127

Creamy Cauliflower Soup 128

Tomato Basil Soup 130

Coconut Curry Lentil Soup 131

Miso Mushroom Soup 132

Detox Lentil Soup 134

Creamy Cauliflower Soup 135

Tomato Basil Soup 136

Coconut Curry Lentil Soup 138

SMOOTHIES RECIPES 140

Green Goddess Smoothie 140

Berry Blast Smoothie 141

Tropical Sunshine Smoothie 142

Chocolate Peanut Butter Protein Smoothie 142

Detox Green Smoothie 143

Berry Protein Smoothie 144

Pineapple Coconut Smoothie 145

Mango Avocado Smoothie 146

Green Tea Smoothie 147

Chocolate Banana Peanut Butter Smoothie 148

Green Detox Smoothie 149

Berry Blast Smoothie 150

Tropical Paradise Smoothie 151

Creamy Peanut Butter Smoothie 152

Chia Berry Smoothie Bowl 153

Green Power Smoothie 154

Creamy Peanut Butter Banana Smoothie 155

Turmeric Mango Smoothie 156

Antioxidant Superfood Smoothie 157

MEAL PLAN 159

   Day 1 159

   Day 2 159

   Day 3 159

   Day 4 159

   Day 5 159

   Day 6 160

   Day 7 160

   Day 8 160

   Day 9 160

   Day 10 160

   Day 11 160

   Day 12 161

   Day 13 161

Day 14 161

Day 15 161

Day 16 161

Day 17 162

Day 18 162

Day 19 162

Day 20 162

Day 21 162

CONCLUSION 163

INTRODUCTION

Dear Reader, Welcome to the world of the EPI Diet Food List for Beginners! If you're holding this book, chances are you're either embarking on a journey to manage Exocrine Pancreatic Insufficiency (EPI) or supporting someone who is. First off, let me extend a virtual high-five to you for taking this step. I know, managing dietary restrictions might not sound like the most thrilling adventure, but trust me, we're about to make it as exciting as a foodie's dream come true.

Now, before we dive into the nitty-gritty of the EPI Diet, let's address the elephant in the room. Dealing with a condition like EPI isn't a walk in the park. It's more like a roller coaster ride with unexpected loops and twists, where the only constant is the queasy feeling in your stomach. I get it. The frustration of not being able to enjoy your favorite foods without worrying about the aftermath can be downright disheartening. But fear not, my friend, for you are not alone on this gastronomic adventure.

You see, I've been there, stomach gurgling like a malfunctioning symphony orchestra, desperately scouring the internet for a lifeline in the form of digestible meals. And let me tell you, the struggle was real. That's why I poured my heart, soul, and probably a few drops of sweat into crafting this book. Consider it your roadmap through the culinary labyrinth of EPI management. But hey, don't worry, I promise there are no Minotaur's lurking in these pages just plenty of delicious recipes and helpful tips to guide you along the way.

In this book, we'll embark on a journey of discovery together. We'll unravel the mysteries of the EPI Diet, decode its secrets, and uncover a treasure trove of delectable dishes that won't leave you clutching your stomach in agony. From understanding the fundamentals of the EPI Diet to whipping up mouthwatering meals that even your non-EPI friends will envy, we've got you covered.

But before we delve into the meat (pun intended) of the book, let me take a moment to express my heartfelt empathy for what you're going through. I know it's not easy navigating the murky waters of dietary restrictions, especially when it feels like everyone else is feasting on forbidden fruits (figuratively speaking, of course). But trust me when I say this: you are stronger than you think, and with the right tools and mindset, you can conquer anything even a stubborn pancreas.

So, my fellow EPI warrior, let's embark on this culinary odyssey together. Consider me your trusty sidekick, guiding you through the culinary wilderness with wit, wisdom, and maybe a sprinkle of sarcasm for good measure. Together, we'll turn your kitchen into a battleground of flavor, where every meal is a victory against digestive woes and every bite a celebration of resilience.

Buckle up, my friend. The journey ahead may be bumpy, but with a dash of determination and a pinch of humor, we'll navigate through it with style. So grab your spatula, dust off your apron, and let's get cooking!

Bon appétit!

Warm regards,

UNDERSTANDING THE EPI DIET

As a nutritionist specializing in gastrointestinal health, I've encountered numerous individuals grappling with the challenges of managing Exocrine Pancreatic Insufficiency (EPI). In this chapter, we'll delve into the intricacies of the EPI Diet, exploring its fundamental principles, its significance in EPI management, and the overarching goals it aims to achieve.

What is EPI?

EPI, short for Exocrine Pancreatic Insufficiency, is a condition characterized by the inadequate production and secretion of digestive enzymes by the pancreas. These enzymes, including lipase, protease, and amylase, play crucial roles in breaking down fats, proteins, and carbohydrates from food, facilitating their absorption in the small intestine.

The root cause of EPI varies, ranging from pancreatic diseases such as chronic pancreatitis, cystic fibrosis, and pancreatic cancer to conditions affecting the pancreatic ducts or surrounding tissues. Regardless of the underlying cause, the hallmark of EPI remains consistent—an impaired ability to digest and absorb nutrients properly, leading to a range of symptoms including abdominal discomfort, diarrhea, weight loss, and nutritional deficiencies.

Understanding the mechanisms behind EPI is pivotal in devising effective management strategies, with dietary modifications playing a central role in optimizing nutrient absorption and minimizing symptoms. While EPI necessitates medical intervention, including enzyme replacement therapy (ERT), dietary adjustments complement these treatments, empowering individuals to take charge of their health and enhance their quality of life.

Importance of Diet in EPI Management

The importance of diet in managing EPI cannot be overstated. Given the compromised digestive function inherent in this condition, dietary choices profoundly influence symptom severity, nutrient absorption, and overall well-being. By tailoring dietary intake to accommodate the unique needs of individuals with EPI, we can mitigate symptoms, promote optimal nutrition, and enhance quality of life.

One of the primary challenges faced by individuals with EPI is the malabsorption of fats, resulting in steatorrhea (excess fat in stools) and deficiencies in fat-soluble vitamins such as A, D, E, and K. Consequently, dietary recommendations for EPI focus on optimizing fat digestion and absorption while ensuring adequate intake of essential nutrients.

To achieve this, the EPI Diet emphasizes the consumption of easily digestible fats, such as medium-chain triglycerides (MCTs) found in coconut oil, as well as lean proteins and complex carbohydrates. Additionally, spreading fat intake throughout the day and pairing fatty foods with enzyme supplements can enhance fat absorption and reduce gastrointestinal symptoms.

In addition to fat malabsorption, individuals with EPI may also experience challenges digesting proteins and carbohydrates, necessitating further dietary modifications. Incorporating enzyme supplements with meals rich in protein and carbohydrates can facilitate their digestion and absorption, alleviating symptoms such as bloating, gas, and abdominal discomfort.

Furthermore, dietary fiber, while essential for digestive health, may exacerbate symptoms in individuals with EPI due to its bulking effect and potential to ferment in the gut, leading to gas and bloating. Therefore, selecting soluble fiber sources such as oats, barley, and fruits, and gradually increasing fiber intake while monitoring symptoms is advisable.

Beyond macronutrient composition, attention should also be paid to micronutrient adequacy, particularly in light of potential deficiencies associated with EPI. Supplementation with fat-soluble vitamins, pancreatic enzyme replacement therapy (PERT), and adherence to a nutrient-rich diet can help address these deficiencies and support overall health.

Goals of the EPI Diet

The overarching goals of the EPI Diet encompass symptom management, nutritional optimization, and lifestyle adaptation. By adhering to these goals, individuals with EPI can achieve improved symptom control, enhanced nutrient absorption, and a better quality of life.

First and foremost, the EPI Diet aims to alleviate gastrointestinal symptoms associated with EPI, including abdominal pain, bloating, diarrhea, and steatorrhea. This is achieved through strategic dietary modifications that minimize the burden on the compromised pancreas, such as reducing fat intake, optimizing enzyme supplementation, and avoiding trigger foods that exacerbate symptoms.

Simultaneously, the EPI Diet endeavors to optimize nutritional intake, ensuring individuals with EPI receive adequate nutrients despite impaired digestion and absorption. This involves selecting nutrient-dense foods that are easily digestible and well tolerated, as well as supplementing with vitamins and minerals as needed to address deficiencies.

Moreover, the EPI Diet seeks to empower individuals with EPI to make informed dietary choices that support their health and well-being in the long term. This includes educating them about the principles of the EPI Diet, providing practical guidance on meal planning and preparation, and fostering a supportive environment conducive to dietary adherence.

Ultimately, the goal of the EPI Diet is to improve overall quality of life for individuals with EPI, enabling them to manage their condition effectively, enjoy a varied and satisfying diet, and lead fulfilling lives free from the constraints of digestive distress.

In the subsequent chapters, we'll explore these concepts in greater detail, offering practical tips, delicious recipes, and personalized meal plans to guide you on your journey towards optimal health with EPI.

As we embark on this culinary adventure together, remember that you are not alone. With the right knowledge, support, and a dash of creativity in the kitchen, managing EPI can be not just manageable, but empowering. So let's roll up our sleeves, sharpen our knives, and dive into the delicious world of the EPI Diet.

FUNDAMENTALS OF THE EPI DIET

Navigating the dietary landscape with Exocrine Pancreatic Insufficiency (EPI) requires a blend of knowledge, strategy, and culinary creativity. In this chapter, we'll delve into the core principles of the EPI Diet, equipping you with the tools and insights necessary to optimize your nutritional intake and manage your condition effectively.

Overview of the EPI Diet

The EPI Diet is a tailored approach to eating designed to support individuals with EPI in managing their symptoms and optimizing nutrient absorption. Unlike one-size-fits-all diet plans, the EPI Diet recognizes the unique challenges posed by impaired pancreatic function and seeks to address them through strategic dietary modifications.

At its core, the EPI Diet emphasizes the consumption of nutrient-dense foods that are easily digestible and well tolerated, while minimizing the intake of foods that may exacerbate symptoms or hinder nutrient absorption. By aligning dietary choices with the specific needs of individuals with EPI, the EPI Diet aims to alleviate gastrointestinal distress, prevent nutrient deficiencies, and enhance overall well-being.

Key Principles and Guidelines

Central to the EPI Diet are several key principles and guidelines that serve as the foundation for dietary management of EPI:

- **Moderation and Balance**: The EPI Diet encourages a balanced approach to eating, with a focus on consuming a variety of nutrient-rich foods from all food groups. By striking a balance between macronutrients (carbohydrates, proteins, and fats) and micronutrients (vitamins and minerals), individuals with EPI can meet their nutritional needs while minimizing digestive discomfort.

- **Optimize Fat Digestion**: Given the impaired ability to digest fats in individuals with EPI, optimizing fat digestion is paramount. This involves selecting easily digestible fats, such as medium-chain triglycerides (MCTs) found in coconut oil, and pairing fatty foods with enzyme supplements to facilitate absorption.

- **Enhance Protein and Carbohydrate Digestion**: Protein and carbohydrate digestion may also be compromised in individuals with EPI, necessitating attention to enzyme supplementation and dietary choices. Consuming enzyme supplements with meals rich in proteins and carbohydrates can aid digestion and reduce symptoms such as bloating and gas.

- **Mindful Fiber Intake**: While dietary fiber is essential for digestive health, excessive intake may exacerbate symptoms in individuals with EPI. Therefore, the EPI Diet recommends selecting soluble fiber sources such as oats, barley, and fruits, and gradually increasing fiber intake while monitoring symptoms.

- **Nutrient Supplementation**: In cases where nutrient deficiencies are present, supplementation may be necessary to address gaps in intake and support overall health. Fat-soluble vitamins (A, D, E, and K) are of particular concern due to malabsorption in individuals with EPI, necessitating supplementation to prevent deficiencies.

- **Regular Monitoring and Adjustment**: The EPI Diet is not static but rather dynamic, requiring regular monitoring and adjustment based on individual needs and response to dietary interventions. By keeping track of symptoms, nutrient intake, and overall well-being, individuals with EPI can fine-tune their dietary approach to achieve optimal outcomes.

Foods to Include and Avoid

When it comes to selecting foods on the EPI Diet, there are certain categories to prioritize and others to limit or avoid:

Foods to Include:
- Lean proteins: Skinless poultry, fish, tofu, legumes
- Complex carbohydrates: Whole grains, fruits, vegetables
- Healthy fats: Olive oil, avocado, nuts, seeds
- Enzyme-rich foods: Papaya, pineapple, kiwi
- Nutrient-dense foods: Eggs, dairy products, fortified cereals

Foods to Limit or Avoid:
- High-fat foods: Fried foods, fatty cuts of meat, creamy sauces
- High-fiber foods: Raw vegetables, bran cereals, beans
- Gas-producing foods: Cruciferous vegetables, beans, carbonated beverages
- Highly processed foods: Packaged snacks, sugary desserts, fast food
- Trigger foods: Spicy foods, caffeine, alcohol

By prioritizing nutrient-dense, easily digestible foods and minimizing intake of foods that may exacerbate symptoms, individuals with EPI can optimize their dietary intake and support digestive health.

Importance of Nutrient Absorption

Optimal nutrient absorption is essential for overall health and well-being, yet it can be compromised in individuals with EPI due to impaired pancreatic function. The consequences of malabsorption extend beyond gastrointestinal discomfort to encompass nutrient deficiencies, impaired immune function, and reduced quality of life.

By adhering to the principles of the EPI Diet and prioritizing nutrient-rich, easily digestible foods, individuals with EPI can enhance their ability to absorb essential nutrients and mitigate the risk of deficiencies. Additionally, supplementation with pancreatic enzyme replacement therapy (PERT) can further support digestion and absorption, ensuring adequate nutrient intake despite pancreatic insufficiency.

Regular monitoring of nutritional status, including blood tests to assess nutrient levels, is essential for identifying deficiencies early and implementing appropriate interventions. By working closely with healthcare providers and registered dietitians, individuals with EPI can develop personalized dietary plans tailored to their unique needs and goals.

In the subsequent chapters, we'll delve deeper into the practical aspects of implementing the EPI Diet, including meal planning, recipe modification, and lifestyle adjustments. By equipping yourself with knowledge and strategies for managing EPI through diet, you can take control of your health and optimize your well-being.

Until then, remember that you are not alone on this journey. With the right support, guidance, and determination, managing EPI can be not just manageable, but empowering. So let's embark on this culinary adventure together, one delicious meal at a time.

GETTING STARTED WITH THE EPI DIET

Embarking on the journey of managing Exocrine Pancreatic Insufficiency (EPI) through dietary modifications can feel daunting at first. However, with the right tools and strategies in place, transitioning to the EPI Diet can become a seamless and empowering experience. In this chapter, we'll explore essential steps to kick start your journey on the EPI Diet, including meal planning, shopping tips for EPI-friendly foods, and meal prep and cooking techniques.

Planning Your Meals

Meal planning is a cornerstone of successful dietary management, particularly for individuals with EPI. By thoughtfully selecting ingredients and designing balanced meals ahead of time, you can streamline your grocery shopping, optimize nutrient intake, and minimize digestive discomfort. Here are some tips to help you get started with meal planning for the EPI Diet:

- **Prioritize Nutrient-Dense Foods**: Focus on incorporating a variety of nutrient-dense foods into your meals, including lean proteins, complex carbohydrates, healthy fats, and plenty of fruits and vegetables. Aim to include a source of protein, a serving of carbohydrates, and a variety of colorful vegetables in each meal to ensure a balanced nutrient profile.
- **Consider Portion Sizes**: Pay attention to portion sizes when planning your meals, especially when it comes to high-fat or high-fiber foods that may be more challenging to digest. Opt for

smaller, more frequent meals throughout the day to help manage symptoms and prevent discomfort.
- **Include Enzyme-Rich Foods**: Incorporate enzyme-rich foods such as papaya, pineapple, and kiwi into your meals to support digestion. These fruits contain natural enzymes that can aid in the breakdown of fats, proteins, and carbohydrates, helping to alleviate symptoms associated with EPI.
- **Experiment with Recipe Modifications**: Get creative in the kitchen by experimenting with recipe modifications to make them more EPI-friendly. For example, you can reduce the amount of oil or butter called for in recipes, substitute high-fiber ingredients with lower-fiber alternatives, or swap out ingredients that trigger symptoms for more tolerable options.

Shopping Tips for EPI-Friendly Foods

Navigating the grocery store aisles can be overwhelming, especially when you're following a specialized diet like the EPI Diet. However, with a bit of planning and knowledge, you can make shopping for EPI-friendly foods a breeze. Here are some tips to help you navigate the grocery store and stock up on essentials for the EPI Diet:
- **Stick to the Perimeter**: When shopping for EPI-friendly foods, focus on shopping the perimeter of the grocery store where you'll find fresh produce, lean proteins, dairy products, and whole grains. These whole, minimally processed foods are generally more nutrient-dense and better tolerated by individuals with EPI.
- **Read Labels Carefully**: Take the time to read labels carefully when selecting packaged foods, paying attention to the ingredient

list and nutrition facts panel. Look for foods that are low in fat, moderate in fiber, and free from ingredients that may trigger symptoms such as artificial sweeteners or high-fructose corn syrup.

- **Choose Digestible Fats**: Opt for easily digestible fats such as olive oil, avocado, and nuts, which are rich in monounsaturated and polyunsaturated fats. These fats are less likely to cause digestive distress compared to saturated fats found in processed and fried foods.
- **Stock Up on Enzyme Supplements**: Don't forget to stock up on enzyme supplements to support digestion and nutrient absorption. Choose a high-quality pancreatic enzyme replacement therapy (PERT) prescribed by your healthcare provider and take it as directed with meals containing fat or protein.

Meal Prep and Cooking Techniques

Meal prep is a game-changer when it comes to staying on track with the EPI Diet. By preparing ingredients ahead of time and batch-cooking meals, you can save time, reduce stress, and ensure that you always have EPI-friendly options on hand. Here are some meal prep and cooking techniques to help you get started:

- **Batch Cook Proteins**: Cook a large batch of lean proteins such as chicken breast, fish, or tofu at the beginning of the week and portion them out for easy meal assembly. You can use cooked proteins as the base for salads, stir-fries, wraps, or grain bowls throughout the week.

- **Prep Fresh Produce**: Wash, chop, and portion out fresh fruits and vegetables ahead of time to make meal assembly a breeze. Store prepped produce in airtight containers or resalable bags in the refrigerator to keep them fresh and easily accessible for snacking or cooking.
- **Utilize Slow Cooker or Instant Pot**: Embrace the convenience of slow cookers or Instant Pots for hands-off meal preparation. Simply toss in your ingredients, set it, and forget it until mealtime. Slow cooker meals are perfect for busy days when you don't have time to fuss over dinner.
- **Explore Gentle Cooking Methods**: Experiment with gentle cooking methods such as steaming, poaching, or baking to make foods easier to digest. These methods help retain moisture and flavor without adding excess fat or fiber that may exacerbate symptoms.

By incorporating these meal prep and cooking techniques into your routine, you can streamline your meal preparation process, reduce the risk of digestive discomfort, and set yourself up for success on the EPI Diet.

In the subsequent chapters, we'll delve deeper into specific meal planning strategies, recipe ideas, and culinary tips to help you thrive on the EPI Diet. Until then, happy meal planning and bon appétit!

EPI DIET FOOD GROUPS

In the realm of the EPI Diet, selecting the right foods is paramount to managing symptoms and optimizing nutritional intake. In this chapter, we'll explore the various food groups recommended for individuals with Exocrine Pancreatic Insufficiency (EPI), including lean meats, poultry, fish and seafood, plant-based protein sources, healthy fats and oils, essential fatty acids, cooking oils and fats to choose, carbohydrates and fiber, whole grains, fruits and vegetables, and legumes and beans. Each food group plays a unique role in providing essential nutrients while supporting digestive health.

Lean Meats

Lean meats are an excellent source of high-quality protein, essential for muscle maintenance, repair, and overall health. When selecting lean meats for the EPI Diet, opt for cuts with minimal visible fat and trim any excess fat before cooking. Examples of lean meats suitable for individuals with EPI include skinless poultry (such as chicken and turkey breast), lean cuts of beef (such as sirloin or tenderloin), pork loin, and game meats like venison or bison. These protein-rich options provide essential amino acids without overloading the digestive system with excess fat, making them ideal choices for individuals with compromised pancreatic function.

Poultry

Poultry, including chicken and turkey, is a staple in many diets due to its versatility, affordability, and lean protein content. When incorporating poultry into the EPI Diet, opt for skinless cuts and remove any visible fat before cooking. Poultry can be prepared in various ways, including grilling, baking, sautéing, or poaching, providing ample opportunities to experiment with flavors and textures. Additionally, poultry is rich in essential nutrients such as iron, zinc, and B vitamins, which are crucial for overall health and well-being.

Fish and Seafood

Fish and seafood offer a wealth of health benefits, including omega-3 fatty acids, which have been shown to support heart health, brain function, and inflammatory response. When selecting fish and seafood for the EPI Diet, prioritize fatty fish such as salmon, mackerel, trout, and sardines, which are rich sources of omega-3s. Additionally, shellfish like shrimp, crab, and scallops are excellent protein sources with minimal fat content, making them suitable options for individuals with EPI. Incorporating fish and seafood into the EPI Diet provides essential nutrients while promoting digestive health and overall well-being.

Plant-Based Protein Sources

Plant-based protein sources offer a nutrient-rich alternative to animal products and can play a valuable role in the EPI Diet. Legumes, such as beans, lentils, and chickpeas, are excellent sources of protein, fiber, and essential nutrients, making them suitable options for individuals with EPI. Additionally, tofu, tempeh, edamame, and seitan provide plant-based protein options with versatile culinary applications. Incorporating plant-based protein sources into the EPI Diet offers diversity, texture, and flavor while supporting digestive health and overall nutritional adequacy.

Healthy Fats and Oils

Healthy fats and oils are essential components of the EPI Diet, providing essential fatty acids, fat-soluble vitamins, and energy for cellular function. When selecting fats and oils for the EPI Diet, prioritize monounsaturated and polyunsaturated fats, which have been shown to support heart health and overall well-being. Examples of healthy fats and oils suitable for individuals with EPI include olive oil, avocado oil, nuts, seeds, and fatty fish. Incorporating these healthy fats into the EPI Diet offers flavor, satiety, and nutritional benefits while supporting digestive health and overall well-being.

Essential Fatty Acids

Essential fatty acids, including omega-3 and omega-6 fatty acids, play crucial roles in cellular function, inflammation modulation, and brain health. When incorporating essential fatty acids into the EPI Diet, prioritize sources rich in omega-3s, such as fatty fish, flaxseeds, chia seeds, walnuts, and hemp seeds. Additionally, omega-6 fatty acids can be found in sources such as vegetable oils, nuts, and seeds, providing a balance of essential fatty acids necessary for optimal health. Incorporating essential fatty acids into the EPI Diet offers numerous health benefits, including improved cardiovascular health, brain function, and inflammatory response.

Cooking Oils and Fats to Choose

When selecting cooking oils and fats for the EPI Diet, opt for options that are low in saturated fats and high in monounsaturated and polyunsaturated fats. Examples of healthy cooking oils and fats suitable for individuals with EPI include olive oil, avocado oil, canola oil, and grapeseed oil. Additionally, incorporating sources of healthy fats such as nuts, seeds, and fatty fish into cooking and meal preparation can provide flavor, texture, and essential nutrients while supporting digestive health and overall well-being.

Carbohydrates and Fiber

Carbohydrates are a primary source of energy for the body and play a crucial role in supporting overall health and well-being. When selecting carbohydrates for the EPI Diet, prioritize complex carbohydrates rich in fiber, vitamins, and minerals, while minimizing simple carbohydrates and refined sugars. Examples of healthy carbohydrates suitable for individuals with EPI include whole grains, fruits, vegetables, and legumes, which provide sustained energy, satiety, and essential nutrients. Incorporating carbohydrates into the EPI Diet offers numerous health benefits, including improved digestive health, blood sugar control, and overall well-being.

Whole Grains

Whole grains are an essential component of the EPI Diet, providing essential nutrients, dietary fiber, and sustained energy. When selecting whole grains for the EPI Diet, opt for options such as brown rice, quinoa, barley, oats, and whole wheat, which provide fiber, vitamins, minerals, and antioxidants. Additionally, incorporating whole grains into meals and snacks offers texture, flavor, and nutritional benefits while supporting digestive health and overall well-being.

Fruits and Vegetables

Fruits and vegetables are nutritional powerhouses, rich in vitamins, minerals, antioxidants, and fiber. When incorporating fruits and vegetables into the EPI Diet, prioritize a variety of colors and types to maximize nutrient intake and diversity. Examples of fruits and vegetables suitable for individuals with EPI include leafy greens, berries, citrus fruits, cruciferous vegetables, and root vegetables, which provide essential nutrients while supporting digestive health and overall well-being. Incorporating fruits and vegetables into the EPI Diet offers numerous health benefits, including improved digestion, immune function, and overall well-being.

Legumes and Beans

Legumes and beans are versatile plant-based protein sources rich in fiber, vitamins, minerals, and antioxidants. When incorporating legumes and beans into the EPI Diet, opt for options such as lentils, black beans, chickpeas, and kidney beans, which provide protein, fiber, and essential nutrients. Additionally, incorporating legumes and beans into meals and snacks offers texture, flavor, and nutritional benefits while supporting digestive health and overall well-being. Incorporating legumes and beans into the EPI Diet offers numerous health benefits, including improved satiety, blood sugar control, and digestive health.

Incorporating these diverse food groups into the EPI Diet offers numerous health benefits, including improved digestion, nutrient intake, and overall well-being. By prioritizing nutrient-dense, easily digestible foods and minimizing intake of foods that may exacerbate symptoms, individuals with EPI can optimize their dietary intake and support digestive health.

TIPS FOR SUCCESS AND ADDITIONAL RESOURCES

Navigating life with Exocrine Pancreatic Insufficiency (EPI) requires more than just knowing which foods to eat. In this chapter, we'll explore practical tips for adhering to the EPI Diet, strategies for navigating eating out and social situations, techniques for managing digestive symptoms, ways to stay motivated and consistent, and additional resources and support available to individuals with EPI.

Adhering to the EPI Diet can be challenging, especially in the face of social gatherings, tempting restaurant menus, and unexpected digestive symptoms. However, with the right strategies and mindset, you can successfully manage your condition and thrive on the EPI Diet.

Tips for Adhering to the EPI Diet

- **Plan Ahead**: Planning ahead is key to success on the EPI Diet. Take time to plan your meals, snacks, and grocery lists in advance, ensuring you have EPI-friendly options readily available when hunger strikes.
- **Keep a Food Diary**: Keeping a food diary can help you track your dietary intake, identify trigger foods, and monitor symptoms. Note what you eat, when you eat it, and any symptoms experienced afterward to pinpoint patterns and make informed decisions about your diet.
- **Be Prepared**: Always have enzyme supplements on hand when eating meals containing fat or protein. Keep a stash in your purse,

car, or desk drawer to ensure you're prepared for any dining situation.

- **Communicate with Your Healthcare Team**: Stay in regular communication with your healthcare team, including your gastroenterologist, dietitian, and primary care provider. Share any changes in symptoms or dietary challenges you're experiencing to receive personalized guidance and support.

Eating Out and Social Situations

Eating out and social situations can present unique challenges for individuals with EPI. However, with a bit of planning and flexibility, you can navigate these scenarios with ease:

- **Research Menus in Advance**: Before dining out, research restaurant menus online to identify EPI-friendly options. Look for dishes that are grilled, steamed, or baked rather than fried, and ask for sauces and dressings on the side to control fat intake.

- **Communicate with Servers**: Don't hesitate to communicate your dietary needs and preferences with servers when dining out. Ask questions about how dishes are prepared and request modifications as needed to accommodate your EPI Diet.

- **Practice Portion Control**: Practice portion control when dining out by splitting entrees with a dining companion, ordering appetizers or side dishes as your main course, or requesting a to-go box to save leftovers for later.

- **Bring EPI-Friendly Snacks**: When attending social gatherings or events, bring EPI-friendly snacks to ensure you have something to munch on that won't exacerbate symptoms. Portable options like nuts, seeds, dried fruit, and protein bars can be lifesavers in a pinch.

Managing Digestive Symptoms

Managing digestive symptoms is a crucial aspect of living with EPI. While dietary modifications play a central role, there are additional strategies you can employ to alleviate discomfort:

- **Stay Hydrated**: Drink plenty of water throughout the day to stay hydrated and support digestive health. Aim for at least 8-10 glasses of water per day, and consider sipping on herbal teas or infused water for added flavor and hydration.
- **Practice Stress Management**: Stress can exacerbate digestive symptoms in individuals with EPI. Practice stress management techniques such as deep breathing, meditation, yoga, or journaling to promote relaxation and reduce tension in the body.
- **Get Moving**: Regular physical activity can help promote digestion and alleviate symptoms of constipation and bloating. Aim for at least 30 minutes of moderate exercise most days of the week, incorporating activities you enjoy such as walking, swimming, or cycling.
- **Consider Probiotics**: Probiotics may help support digestive health by replenishing beneficial gut bacteria. Talk to your healthcare provider about whether probiotic supplements or fermented foods like yogurt, kefir, and sauerkraut may be beneficial for you.

Staying Motivated and Consistent

Staying motivated and consistent on the EPI Diet can be challenging, especially in the face of setbacks or temptation. Here are some strategies to help you stay on track:

- **Set Realistic Goals**: Set realistic, achievable goals for yourself on the EPI Diet. Break larger goals into smaller, manageable steps, and celebrate your progress along the way.
- **Find Support**: Surround yourself with a supportive network of friends, family, and healthcare professionals who understand your dietary needs and can offer encouragement and guidance when needed.
- **Focus on Progress, Not Perfection**: Remember that perfection is not the goal on the EPI Diet. Instead of striving for perfection, focus on making progress toward your health and wellness goals one day at a time.
- **Practice Self-Care**: Take time for self-care and prioritize activities that nourish your body, mind, and spirit. Whether it's indulging in a relaxing bath, going for a nature walk, or spending time with loved ones, prioritize activities that bring you joy and rejuvenation.

Additional Resources and Support

In addition to the tips and strategies outlined above, there are numerous resources and support systems available to individuals with EPI:

- **Online Communities**: Join online communities and support groups for individuals with EPI to connect with others who understand your experiences and can offer advice, encouragement, and support.

- **Educational Materials**: Seek out educational materials and resources on EPI from reputable sources such as medical organizations, research institutions, and patient advocacy groups. Knowledge is power, and arming yourself with accurate information can empower you to take control of your health.
- **Healthcare Providers**: Consult with your healthcare providers, including your gastroenterologist, dietitian, and primary care provider, for personalized guidance and support tailored to your specific needs and circumstances.
- **Patient Advocacy Groups**: Explore patient advocacy groups and organizations dedicated to supporting individuals with EPI and raising awareness about the condition. These groups may offer educational resources, support services, and opportunities for advocacy and community involvement.

By utilizing these resources and implementing the tips and strategies outlined in this chapter, you can successfully navigate life with EPI and thrive on the EPI Diet. Remember that you are not alone on this journey, and support is available to help you achieve your health and wellness goals.

In the subsequent chapters, we'll delve deeper into specific aspects of the EPI Diet, including meal planning, recipe ideas, and culinary inspiration, to help you put these strategies into practice. Until then, stay motivated, stay consistent, and remember that you have the power to take control of your health and well-being.

BREAKFAST RECIPES

Savory Breakfast Quinoa Bowl

Prep Time: 5 mins

Total Time: 20 mins

Servings: 2 bowls

Ingredients:

- 1 cup quinoa, rinsed
- 2 cups water or low-sodium vegetable broth
- 1 tablespoon olive oil
- 1/2 onion, diced
- 1 bell pepper, diced
- 2 cloves garlic, minced
- 2 cups fresh spinach
- Salt and pepper to taste
- 1 avocado, sliced
- 2 poached eggs (optional)
- Fresh herbs for garnish (e.g., parsley, chives)

Directions:

1. In a medium saucepan, combine quinoa and water or broth. Bring to a boil, then reduce heat to low, cover, and simmer for 15 minutes, or until quinoa is cooked and liquid is absorbed.
2. While quinoa is cooking, heat olive oil in a skillet over medium heat. Add diced onion and bell pepper, and sauté until softened, about 5 minutes. Add minced garlic and cook for an additional minute.

3. Add fresh spinach to the skillet and cook until wilted. Season with salt and pepper to taste.
4. Divide cooked quinoa between two bowls. Top with sautéed vegetables, sliced avocado, and poached eggs (if using).
5. Garnish with fresh herbs and serve hot.

Nutrition Facts (per serving):
- Calories: 395
- Protein: 13g
- Fat: 18g
- Carbohydrates: 50g
- Fiber: 9g

Blueberry Almond Chia Pudding

Prep Time: 5 mins

Total Time: 4 hours (chilling time)

Servings: 2 servings

Ingredients:
- 1/4 cup chia seeds
- 1 cup unsweetened almond milk
- 1/2 teaspoon vanilla extract
- 1 tablespoon maple syrup or honey (optional)
- 1/2 cup fresh blueberries
- 2 tablespoons sliced almonds

Directions:
1. In a mixing bowl, combine chia seeds, almond milk, vanilla extract, and maple syrup or honey (if using). Stir well to combine.

2. Cover the bowl and refrigerate for at least 4 hours or overnight, until the mixture has thickened to a pudding-like consistency.
3. Before serving, stir the chia pudding to redistribute the seeds. Divide the pudding between two serving glasses or bowls.
4. Top each serving with fresh blueberries and sliced almonds.
5. Serve chilled.

Nutrition Facts (per serving):
- Calories: 245
- Protein: 6g
- Fat: 14g
- Carbohydrates: 25g
- Fiber: 10g

Spinach and Feta Omelette

Prep Time: 5 mins

Total Time: 10 mins

Servings: 1 omelette

Ingredients:
- 2 large eggs
- 1 tablespoon water or milk
- Salt and pepper to taste
- 1 teaspoon olive oil
- 1 cup fresh spinach
- 2 tablespoons crumbled feta cheese

Directions:
1. In a small bowl, whisk together eggs, water or milk, salt, and pepper until well combined.

2. Heat olive oil in a non-stick skillet over medium heat. Add fresh spinach and cook until wilted, about 1-2 minutes.
3. Pour the egg mixture into the skillet, tilting the pan to distribute the eggs evenly.
4. Cook the omelette for 2-3 minutes, or until the edges start to set and the bottom is lightly golden.
5. Sprinkle crumbled feta cheese over one half of the omelette. Fold the other half over the filling.
6. Cook for an additional 1-2 minutes, or until the cheese is melted and the eggs are cooked through.
7. Slide the omelette onto a plate and serve hot.

Nutrition Facts (per serving):
- Calories: 250
- Protein: 19g
- Fat: 17g
- Carbohydrates: 3g
- Fiber: 1g

Avocado Toast with Smoked Salmon

Prep Time: 5 mins

Total Time: 10 mins

Servings: 2 slices

Ingredients:
- 2 slices whole grain bread, toasted
- 1 ripe avocado
- Juice of 1/2 lemon
- Salt and pepper to taste

- 2 ounces smoked salmon
- 1 tablespoon capers
- Fresh dill for garnish

Directions:

1. In a small bowl, mash the ripe avocado with lemon juice, salt, and pepper until smooth and creamy.
2. Spread the mashed avocado evenly onto the toasted bread slices.
3. Top each slice with smoked salmon and sprinkle with capers.
4. Garnish with fresh dill leaves.
5. Serve immediately.

Nutrition Facts (per serving):

- Calories: 230
- Protein: 13g
- Fat: 13g
- Carbohydrates: 18g
- Fiber: 6g

Greek Yogurt Parfait with Berries and Granola

Prep Time: 5 mins

Total Time: 5 mins

Servings: 1 parfait

Ingredients:

- 1/2 cup plain Greek yogurt
- 1/4 cup fresh mixed berries (e.g., strawberries, blueberries, raspberries)
- 1/4 cup granola (choose a low-fat, low-sugar option)

- 1 tablespoon honey or maple syrup (optional)

Directions:
1. In a serving glass or bowl, layer Greek yogurt, mixed berries, and granola.
2. Drizzle honey or maple syrup over the top, if desired.
3. Repeat layers until the glass or bowl is filled.
4. Serve immediately as a nutritious and satisfying breakfast option.

Nutrition Facts (per serving):
- Calories: 250
- Protein: 15g
- Fat: 5g
- Carbohydrates: 35g
- Fiber: 5g

Egg and Vegetable Breakfast Burrito

Prep Time: 10 mins

Total Time: 20 mins

Servings: 2 burritos

Ingredients:
- 4 large eggs
- 1/4 cup diced bell peppers (any color)
- 1/4 cup diced onions
- 1/4 cup diced tomatoes
- 1/4 cup diced mushrooms
- 2 whole grain tortillas
- Salt and pepper to taste

- 1/4 cup shredded cheese (optional)
- Salsa and avocado slices for serving

Directions:
1. In a mixing bowl, whisk the eggs until well beaten. Season with salt and pepper to taste.
2. Heat a non-stick skillet over medium heat. Add diced bell peppers, onions, tomatoes, and mushrooms, and sauté until softened, about 5 minutes.
3. Pour the beaten eggs over the cooked vegetables in the skillet. Cook, stirring occasionally, until the eggs are set and scrambled.
4. Divide the scrambled eggs and vegetable mixture between two whole grain tortillas. Sprinkle shredded cheese on top if desired.
5. Roll up the tortillas to form burritos, folding in the sides as you go.
6. Serve the breakfast burritos with salsa and avocado slices on the side.

Nutrition Facts (per serving):
- Calories: 320
- Protein: 17g
- Fat: 14g
- Carbohydrates: 30g
- Fiber: 6g

Quinoa Breakfast Porridge

Prep Time: 5 mins

Total Time: 15 mins

Servings: 2 bowls

Ingredients:

- 1/2 cup quinoa, rinsed
- 1 cup almond milk
- 1/2 teaspoon ground cinnamon
- 1 tablespoon maple syrup or honey
- 1/4 cup chopped nuts (e.g., almonds, walnuts)
- Fresh fruit for topping (e.g., berries, sliced banana)

Directions:

1. In a saucepan, combine quinoa and almond milk. Bring to a boil, then reduce heat to low, cover, and simmer for 10-12 minutes, or until quinoa is cooked and liquid is absorbed.
2. Stir in ground cinnamon and maple syrup or honey. Cook for an additional 2-3 minutes, stirring occasionally.
3. Divide the quinoa porridge between two bowls. Top with chopped nuts and fresh fruit.
4. Serve hot and enjoy!

Nutrition Facts (per serving):

- Calories: 320
- Protein: 9g
- Fat: 12g
- Carbohydrates: 45g
- Fiber: 6g

Sweet Potato and Black Bean Breakfast Hash

Prep Time: 10 mins

Total Time: 30 mins

Servings: 2 servings

Ingredients:

- 1 large sweet potato, diced
- 1/2 onion, diced
- 1 bell pepper, diced
- 1 cup cooked black beans
- 1 teaspoon ground cumin
- 1/2 teaspoon smoked paprika
- Salt and pepper to taste
- 2 eggs
- Fresh cilantro for garnish

Directions:

1. Heat olive oil in a skillet over medium heat. Add diced sweet potato and cook until tender, about 10-12 minutes.
2. Add diced onion and bell pepper to the skillet and cook until softened, about 5 minutes.
3. Stir in cooked black beans, ground cumin, smoked paprika, salt, and pepper. Cook for an additional 2-3 minutes, until heated through.
4. Create two wells in the hash mixture and crack an egg into each well.
5. Cover the skillet and cook for 5-7 minutes, or until the eggs are cooked to your desired doneness.
6. Garnish with fresh cilantro and serve hot.

Nutrition Facts (per serving):
- Calories: 320
- Protein: 15g
- Fat: 10g
- Carbohydrates: 45g
- Fiber: 10g

Coconut Chia Seed Pudding

Prep Time: 5 mins

Total Time: 4 hours (chilling time)

Servings: 2 servings

Ingredients:
- 1/4 cup chia seeds
- 1 cup coconut milk
- 1 tablespoon maple syrup or honey (optional)
- 1/2 teaspoon vanilla extract
- 1/4 cup toasted coconut flakes

Directions:
1. In a mixing bowl, combine chia seeds, coconut milk, maple syrup or honey (if using), and vanilla extract. Stir well to combine.
2. Cover the bowl and refrigerate for at least 4 hours or overnight, until the mixture has thickened to a pudding-like consistency.
3. Before serving, stir the chia pudding to redistribute the seeds. Divide the pudding between two serving glasses or bowls.
4. Top each serving with toasted coconut flakes.
5. Serve chilled and enjoy!

Nutrition Facts (per serving):
- Calories: 280
- Protein: 5g
- Fat: 22g
- Carbohydrates: 20g
- Fiber: 10g

Quinoa Breakfast Bowl

Prep Time: 5 mins

Total Time: 20 mins

Servings: 2 bowls

Ingredients:
- 1/2 cup quinoa, rinsed
- 1 cup water or vegetable broth
- 1 tablespoon olive oil
- 1/2 onion, diced
- 1 bell pepper, diced
- 2 cups fresh spinach
- 4 large eggs
- Salt and pepper to taste
- Fresh herbs for garnish (e.g., parsley, chives)

Directions:
1. In a saucepan, bring water or vegetable broth to a boil. Add quinoa, reduce heat to low, cover, and simmer for 15 minutes, or until quinoa is cooked and liquid is absorbed.

2. While quinoa is cooking, heat olive oil in a skillet over medium heat. Add diced onion and bell pepper, and sauté until softened, about 5 minutes.
3. Add fresh spinach to the skillet and cook until wilted. Season with salt and pepper to taste.
4. In a separate non-stick skillet, fry the eggs to your desired doneness.
5. Divide cooked quinoa between two bowls. Top with sautéed vegetables and fried eggs.
6. Garnish with fresh herbs and serve hot.

Nutrition Facts (per serving):
- Calories: 320
- Protein: 17g
- Fat: 14g
- Carbohydrates: 30g
- Fiber: 6g

Smoked Salmon and Avocado Toast

Prep Time: 5 mins

Total Time: 10 mins

Servings: 2 slices

Ingredients:
- 2 slices whole grain bread, toasted
- 1 ripe avocado
- Juice of 1/2 lemon
- Salt and pepper to taste
- 2 ounces smoked salmon

- 2 tablespoons capers

Directions:

1. In a small bowl, mash the ripe avocado with lemon juice, salt, and pepper until smooth and creamy.
2. Spread the mashed avocado evenly onto the toasted bread slices.
3. Top each slice with smoked salmon and sprinkle with capers.
4. Serve immediately.

Nutrition Facts (per serving):

- Calories: 280
- Protein: 15g
- Fat: 12g
- Carbohydrates: 30g
- Fiber: 7g

Greek Yogurt Parfait

Prep Time: 5 mins

Total Time: 5 mins

Servings: 2 servings

Ingredients:

- 1 cup plain Greek yogurt
- 1/2 cup fresh mixed berries (e.g., strawberries, blueberries, raspberries)
- 1/4 cup granola (choose a low-fat, low-sugar option)
- 1 tablespoon honey or maple syrup (optional)

Directions:

1. In a serving glass or bowl, layer Greek yogurt, mixed berries, and granola.
2. Drizzle honey or maple syrup over the top, if desired.
3. Serve immediately.

Nutrition Facts (per serving):
- Calories: 250
- Protein: 15g
- Fat: 5g
- Carbohydrates: 35g
- Fiber: 5g

Spinach and Feta Omelette

Prep Time: 5 mins

Total Time: 10 mins

Servings: 1 omelette

Ingredients:
- 2 large eggs
- 1 tablespoon water or milk
- Salt and pepper to taste
- 1 teaspoon olive oil
- 1 cup fresh spinach
- 2 tablespoons crumbled feta cheese

Directions:
1. In a small bowl, whisk together eggs, water or milk, salt, and pepper until well combined.
2. Heat olive oil in a non-stick skillet over medium heat. Add fresh spinach and cook until wilted, about 1-2 minutes.

3. Pour the egg mixture into the skillet, tilting the pan to distribute the eggs evenly.
4. Cook the omelette for 2-3 minutes, or until the edges start to set and the bottom is lightly golden.
5. Sprinkle crumbled feta cheese over one half of the omelette. Fold the other half over the filling.
6. Cook for an additional 1-2 minutes, or until the cheese is melted and the eggs are cooked through.
7. Slide the omelette onto a plate and serve hot.

Nutrition Facts (per serving):
- Calories: 280
- Protein: 19g
- Fat: 17g
- Carbohydrates: 3g
- Fiber: 1g

Blueberry Almond Chia Pudding

Prep Time: 5 mins

Total Time: 4 hours (chilling time)

Servings: 2 servings

Ingredients:
- 1/4 cup chia seeds
- 1 cup unsweetened almond milk
- 1/2 teaspoon vanilla extract
- 1 tablespoon maple syrup or honey (optional)
- 1/2 cup fresh blueberries
- 2 tablespoons sliced almonds

Directions:
1. In a mixing bowl, combine chia seeds, almond milk, vanilla extract, and maple syrup or honey (if using). Stir well to combine.
2. Cover the bowl and refrigerate for at least 4 hours or overnight, until the mixture has thickened to a pudding-like consistency.
3. Before serving, stir the chia pudding to redistribute the seeds. Divide the pudding between two serving glasses or bowls.
4. Top each serving with fresh blueberries and sliced almonds.
5. Serve chilled.

Nutrition Facts (per serving):
- Calories: 245
- Protein: 6g
- Fat: 14g
- Carbohydrates: 25g
- Fiber: 10g

Spinach and Mushroom Breakfast Frittata

Prep Time: 10 mins

Total Time: 25 mins

Servings: 4 servings

Ingredients:
- 6 large eggs
- 1/4 cup milk (or dairy-free alternative)
- Salt and pepper to taste
- 1 tablespoon olive oil
- 1/2 onion, diced

- 1 cup sliced mushrooms
- 2 cups fresh spinach
- 1/4 cup shredded cheese (optional)

Directions:
1. Preheat your oven to 350°F (175°C).
2. In a mixing bowl, whisk together eggs, milk, salt, and pepper until well combined.
3. Heat olive oil in an oven-safe skillet over medium heat. Add diced onion and sliced mushrooms, and cook until softened, about 5 minutes.
4. Add fresh spinach to the skillet and cook until wilted.
5. Pour the egg mixture over the cooked vegetables in the skillet. Stir gently to distribute the ingredients evenly.
6. Cook for 2-3 minutes, or until the edges start to set.
7. Sprinkle shredded cheese (if using) over the top of the frittata.
8. Transfer the skillet to the preheated oven and bake for 10-12 minutes, or until the eggs are set and the top is golden brown.
9. Remove from the oven and let cool for a few minutes before slicing and serving.

Nutrition Facts (per serving):
- Calories: 180
- Protein: 12g
- Fat: 11g
- Carbohydrates: 6g
- Fiber: 1g

Overnight Oats with Berries and Almonds

Prep Time: 5 mins

Total Time: 8 hours (overnight chilling)

Servings: 2 servings

Ingredients:
- 1 cup old-fashioned rolled oats
- 1 cup almond milk (or dairy-free alternative)
- 1 tablespoon chia seeds
- 1/2 teaspoon vanilla extract
- 1 tablespoon maple syrup or honey
- 1/2 cup mixed berries (e.g., strawberries, blueberries, raspberries)
- 2 tablespoons sliced almonds

Directions:
1. In a mixing bowl or jar, combine rolled oats, almond milk, chia seeds, vanilla extract, and maple syrup or honey. Stir well to combine.
2. Cover the bowl or jar and refrigerate overnight, or for at least 8 hours.
3. Before serving, stir the overnight oats to mix well. If the mixture is too thick, you can add a splash of almond milk to reach your desired consistency.
4. Divide the overnight oats between two serving bowls.
5. Top each serving with mixed berries and sliced almonds.
6. Serve chilled and enjoy!

Nutrition Facts (per serving):
- Calories: 300

- Protein: 9g
- Fat: 12g
- Carbohydrates: 40g
- Fiber: 8g

Turkey and Vegetable Breakfast Hash

Prep Time: 10 mins

Total Time: 25 mins

Servings: 2 servings

Ingredients:

- 2 tablespoons olive oil
- 1/2 onion, diced
- 1 bell pepper, diced
- 2 cups diced sweet potatoes
- 8 ounces cooked turkey breast, diced
- Salt and pepper to taste
- Fresh parsley for garnish

Directions:

1. Heat olive oil in a skillet over medium heat. Add diced onion and bell pepper, and cook until softened, about 5 minutes.
2. Add diced sweet potatoes to the skillet and cook until tender, about 10-12 minutes.
3. Stir in diced turkey breast and cook until heated through.
4. Season with salt and pepper to taste.
5. Divide the turkey and vegetable hash between two serving plates.
6. Garnish with fresh parsley and serve hot.

Nutrition Facts (per serving):
- Calories: 320
- Protein: 25g
- Fat: 10g
- Carbohydrates: 30g
- Fiber: 6g

Green Breakfast Smoothie Bowl

Prep Time: 5 mins

Total Time: 5 mins

Servings: 1 bowl

Ingredients:
- 1 ripe banana, frozen
- 1 cup fresh spinach
- 1/2 cup frozen pineapple chunks
- 1/2 cup almond milk (or dairy-free alternative)
- 1 tablespoon chia seeds
- 2 tablespoons granola
- Fresh berries for topping

Directions:
1. In a blender, combine frozen banana, fresh spinach, frozen pineapple chunks, almond milk, and chia seeds. Blend until smooth and creamy.
2. Pour the smoothie into a serving bowl.
3. Top with granola and fresh berries.
4. Serve immediately and enjoy!

Nutrition Facts (per serving):

- Calories: 300
- Protein: 7g
- Fat: 10g
- Carbohydrates: 50g
- Fiber: 10g

Avocado and Tomato Breakfast Toast

Prep Time: 5 mins

Total Time: 5 mins

Servings: 2 slices

Ingredients:

- 2 slices whole grain bread, toasted
- 1 ripe avocado
- 1 tomato, sliced
- Salt and pepper to taste
- Fresh basil leaves for garnish

Directions:

1. Mash the ripe avocado in a small bowl. Season with salt and pepper to taste.
2. Spread the mashed avocado evenly onto the toasted bread slices.
3. Top each slice with sliced tomatoes.
4. Garnish with fresh basil leaves.
5. Serve immediately.

Nutrition Facts (per serving):

- Calories: 200
- Protein: 5g

- Fat: 10g
- Carbohydrates: 25g
- Fiber: 8g

SNACKS RECIPES

Chia Seed Pudding

Prep Time: 5 mins

Total Time: 4 hours (chilling time)

Servings: 2 servings

Ingredients:

- 1/4 cup chia seeds
- 1 cup almond milk (or dairy-free alternative)
- 1 tablespoon maple syrup or honey (optional)
- 1/2 teaspoon vanilla extract
- Fresh fruit for topping (e.g., berries, sliced banana)

Directions:

1. In a mixing bowl, combine chia seeds, almond milk, maple syrup or honey (if using), and vanilla extract. Stir well to combine.
2. Cover the bowl and refrigerate for at least 4 hours or overnight, until the mixture has thickened to a pudding-like consistency.
3. Before serving, stir the chia pudding to redistribute the seeds. Divide the pudding between two serving glasses or bowls.
4. Top each serving with fresh fruit.
5. Serve chilled and enjoy!

Nutrition Facts (per serving):

- Calories: 150
- Protein: 5g
- Fat: 8g

- Carbohydrates: 16g
- Fiber: 10g

Apple and Peanut Butter Slices

Prep Time: 5 mins

Total Time: 5 mins

Servings: 2 servings

Ingredients:

- 1 apple, sliced
- 2 tablespoons peanut butter (or almond butter)
- 1 tablespoon honey (optional)
- 1 tablespoon chopped nuts (e.g., almonds, walnuts)

Directions:

1. Arrange the apple slices on a plate or serving dish.
2. Spread peanut butter over each apple slice.
3. Drizzle with honey (if using) and sprinkle with chopped nuts.
4. Serve immediately and enjoy!

Nutrition Facts (per serving):

- Calories: 200
- Protein: 5g
- Fat: 12g
- Carbohydrates: 20g
- Fiber: 4g

Greek Yogurt with Berries and Honey

Prep Time: 5 mins

Total Time: 5 mins

Servings: 2 servings

Ingredients:

- 1 cup plain Greek yogurt
- 1/2 cup mixed berries (e.g., strawberries, blueberries, raspberries)
- 2 tablespoons honey
- 2 tablespoons granola (optional)

Directions:

1. Divide the Greek yogurt between two serving bowls.
2. Top each bowl with mixed berries.
3. Drizzle honey over the berries.
4. Optionally, sprinkle granola over the top for added crunch.
5. Serve immediately and enjoy!

Nutrition Facts (per serving):

- Calories: 200
- Protein: 15g
- Fat: 4g
- Carbohydrates: 30g
- Fiber: 2g

Vegetable Sticks with Hummus

Prep Time: 10 mins

Total Time: 10 mins

Servings: 2 servings

Ingredients:

- Assorted vegetable sticks (e.g., carrots, cucumbers, bell peppers)
- 1/2 cup hummus

Directions:
1. Wash and cut assorted vegetables into sticks.
2. Arrange the vegetable sticks on a serving plate.
3. Serve with hummus for dipping.
4. Enjoy this crunchy and satisfying snack!

Nutrition Facts (per serving):
- Calories: 150
- Protein: 5g
- Fat: 8g
- Carbohydrates: 15g
- Fiber: 6g

Trail Mix

Prep Time: 5 mins
Total Time: 5 mins
Servings: 2 servings

Ingredients:
- 1/4 cup almonds
- 1/4 cup cashews
- 1/4 cup dried cranberries
- 1/4 cup pumpkin seeds
- 1/4 cup dark chocolate chips

Directions:
1. In a mixing bowl, combine all the ingredients.

2. Toss well to mix.
3. Divide the trail mix between two small resalable bags for easy portioning.
4. Enjoy as a convenient and nutritious snack on-the-go!

Nutrition Facts (per serving):
- Calories: 250
- Protein: 8g
- Fat: 15g
- Carbohydrates: 25g
- Fiber: 4g

Energy Balls

Prep Time: 15 mins
Total Time: 15 mins
Servings: 12 balls

Ingredients:
- 1 cup rolled oats
- 1/2 cup almond butter
- 1/4 cup honey or maple syrup
- 1/4 cup ground flaxseed
- 1/4 cup chopped nuts (e.g., almonds, walnuts)
- 1/4 cup dried cranberries or raisins
- 1 teaspoon vanilla extract
- Pinch of salt
- Optional: shredded coconut, cocoa powder for coating

Directions:

1. In a mixing bowl, combine rolled oats, almond butter, honey or maple syrup, ground flaxseed, chopped nuts, dried cranberries or raisins, vanilla extract, and a pinch of salt.
2. Stir well until all ingredients are evenly incorporated.
3. Scoop out tablespoon-sized portions of the mixture and roll into balls using your hands.
4. If desired, roll the energy balls in shredded coconut or cocoa powder for extra flavor.
5. Place the energy balls on a baking sheet lined with parchment paper and chill in the refrigerator for at least 30 minutes before serving.
6. Store leftovers in an airtight container in the refrigerator for up to one week.

Nutrition Facts (per serving - 1 ball):
- Calories: 120
- Protein: 3g
- Fat: 7g
- Carbohydrates: 12g
- Fiber: 2g

Vegetable Sushi Rolls

Prep Time: 20 mins

Total Time: 20 mins

Servings: 4 rolls

Ingredients:
- 4 nori seaweed sheets
- 2 cups cooked quinoa

- 1 small cucumber, julienned
- 1 carrot, julienned
- 1 avocado, sliced
- 1/4 cup pickled ginger (optional)
- 1/4 cup low-sodium soy sauce or tamari
- Wasabi and/or sesame seeds for garnish

Directions:
1. Place a nori seaweed sheet shiny side down on a sushi rolling mat or clean kitchen towel.
2. Spread a thin layer of cooked quinoa evenly over the nori sheet, leaving a 1-inch border at the top edge.
3. Arrange julienned cucumber, carrot, avocado, and pickled ginger in a line across the center of the quinoa.
4. Using the sushi rolling mat or kitchen towel, tightly roll the nori sheet away from you, pressing gently as you roll to seal the ingredients.
5. Use a sharp knife to slice the sushi roll into 6-8 pieces.
6. Serve with low-sodium soy sauce or tamari for dipping, and garnish with wasabi and sesame seeds if desired.
7. Enjoy these nutritious vegetable sushi rolls as a satisfying snack!

Nutrition Facts (per serving - 1 roll):
- Calories: 180
- Protein: 5g
- Fat: 6g
- Carbohydrates: 28g

- Fiber: 6g

Roasted Chickpeas

Prep Time: 5 mins

Total Time: 40 mins

Servings: 4 servings

Ingredients:
- 2 cans (15 ounces each) chickpeas, drained and rinsed
- 2 tablespoons olive oil
- 1 teaspoon ground cumin
- 1 teaspoon paprika
- 1/2 teaspoon garlic powder
- 1/2 teaspoon salt

Directions:
1. Preheat your oven to 400°F (200°C). Line a baking sheet with parchment paper.
2. Pat the rinsed chickpeas dry with a clean kitchen towel or paper towels to remove excess moisture.
3. In a mixing bowl, toss the dried chickpeas with olive oil, ground cumin, paprika, garlic powder, and salt until evenly coated.
4. Spread the seasoned chickpeas in a single layer on the prepared baking sheet.
5. Roast in the preheated oven for 30-40 minutes, stirring halfway through, until the chickpeas are golden brown and crispy.
6. Remove from the oven and let cool before serving.

7. Enjoy these crunchy roasted chickpeas as a nutritious and satisfying snack!

Nutrition Facts (per serving):
- Calories: 220
- Protein: 8g
- Fat: 8g
- Carbohydrates: 28g
- Fiber: 7g

Caprese Skewers

Prep Time: 15 mins

Total Time: 15 mins

Servings: 4 skewers

Ingredients:
- 8 cherry tomatoes
- 8 small fresh mozzarella balls (bocconcini)
- 8 fresh basil leaves
- 1 tablespoon balsamic glaze
- Salt and pepper to taste

Directions:
1. Thread a cherry tomato, a fresh mozzarella ball, and a basil leaf onto each skewer.
2. Repeat until all ingredients are used, making 4 skewers in total.
3. Arrange the skewers on a serving platter.
4. Drizzle balsamic glaze over the skewers and season with salt and pepper to taste.
5. Serve immediately and enjoy this classic Italian-inspired snack!

Nutrition Facts (per serving - 2 skewers):
- Calories: 120
- Protein: 8g
- Fat: 8g
- Carbohydrates: 4g
- Fiber: 1g

Hummus Stuffed Bell Peppers

Prep Time: 10 mins

Total Time: 10 mins

Servings: 4 servings

Ingredients:
- 2 large bell peppers, halved and seeds removed
- 1 cup hummus (store-bought or homemade)
- Paprika and fresh parsley for garnish

Directions:
1. Fill each bell pepper half with a generous scoop of hummus.
2. Sprinkle paprika over the top of the hummus for added flavor and color.
3. Garnish with fresh parsley for a pop of freshness.
4. Serve immediately, or store in the refrigerator until ready to enjoy.
5. These hummus-stuffed bell peppers make a nutritious and satisfying snack option!

Nutrition Facts (per serving - 1 stuffed pepper half):
- Calories: 100
- Protein: 4g

- Fat: 6g
- Carbohydrates: 10g
- Fiber: 4g

Quinoa Salad with Avocado and Chickpeas

Prep Time: 15 mins

Total Time: 20 mins

Servings: 4 servings

Ingredients:

- 1 cup cooked quinoa
- 1 avocado, diced
- 1 can (15 ounces) chickpeas, drained and rinsed
- 1 cup cherry tomatoes, halved
- 1/4 cup chopped fresh cilantro or parsley
- 2 tablespoons olive oil
- 1 tablespoon lemon juice
- Salt and pepper to taste

Directions:

1. In a large mixing bowl, combine cooked quinoa, diced avocado, chickpeas, cherry tomatoes, and chopped cilantro or parsley.
2. Drizzle olive oil and lemon juice over the salad ingredients.
3. Season with salt and pepper to taste.
4. Toss well to combine all the ingredients evenly.
5. Serve immediately or refrigerate until ready to enjoy.
6. This quinoa salad with avocado and chickpeas makes a delicious and satisfying snack option!

Nutrition Facts (per serving):

- Calories: 280
- Protein: 9g
- Fat: 14g
- Carbohydrates: 31g
- Fiber: 9g

Turkey and Cheese Roll-Ups

Prep Time: 10 mins

Total Time: 10 mins

Servings: 2 servings

Ingredients:
- 4 slices turkey breast
- 2 slices cheese (e.g., cheddar, Swiss)
- 1/2 avocado, sliced
- 1/2 cup baby spinach leaves
- Mustard or mayonnaise for spreading (optional)

Directions:
1. Lay the turkey slices flat on a clean work surface.
2. Place a slice of cheese on each turkey slice.
3. Top each slice with avocado slices and baby spinach leaves.
4. If desired, spread mustard or mayonnaise over the ingredients.
5. Roll up each turkey slice tightly to create a roll-up.
6. Secure with toothpicks if necessary.
7. Slice each roll-up into bite-sized pieces.
8. Serve immediately or pack for a convenient snack on-the-go.

Nutrition Facts (per serving):
- Calories: 250

- Protein: 20g
- Fat: 16g
- Carbohydrates: 7g
- Fiber: 4g

Greek Yogurt Parfait

Prep Time: 5 mins

Total Time: 5 mins

Servings: 2 servings

Ingredients:

- 1 cup plain Greek yogurt
- 1/2 cup mixed berries (e.g., strawberries, blueberries, raspberries)
- 1/4 cup granola
- 2 tablespoons honey or maple syrup (optional)

Directions:

1. In two serving glasses or bowls, layer plain Greek yogurt, mixed berries, and granola.
2. Drizzle honey or maple syrup over the top if desired.
3. Repeat the layers until all ingredients are used.
4. Serve immediately and enjoy this nutritious and delicious Greek yogurt parfait!

Nutrition Facts (per serving):

- Calories: 250
- Protein: 18g
- Fat: 6g
- Carbohydrates: 35g

- Fiber: 5g

Zucchini and Carrot Fritters

Prep Time: 15 mins

Total Time: 25 mins

Servings: 4 servings

Ingredients:
- 1 medium zucchini, grated
- 1 medium carrot, grated
- 2 eggs
- 1/4 cup whole wheat flour or almond flour
- 2 tablespoons grated Parmesan cheese
- 2 tablespoons chopped fresh parsley or cilantro
- Salt and pepper to taste
- Olive oil for cooking

Directions:
1. In a large mixing bowl, combine grated zucchini, grated carrot, eggs, whole wheat flour or almond flour, grated Parmesan cheese, chopped fresh parsley or cilantro, salt, and pepper.
2. Stir well until all ingredients are evenly combined.
3. Heat olive oil in a non-stick skillet over medium heat.
4. Scoop out tablespoon-sized portions of the fritter mixture and drop onto the skillet.
5. Flatten each portion with a spatula to form a fritter.
6. Cook for 3-4 minutes on each side, or until golden brown and cooked through.
7. Remove from the skillet and drain on paper towels.

8. Serve the zucchini and carrot fritters warm or at room temperature.
9. These fritters can be enjoyed on their own or served with a dollop of Greek yogurt or hummus for dipping.

Nutrition Facts (per serving):
- Calories: 150
- Protein: 7g
- Fat: 8g
- Carbohydrates: 12g
- Fiber: 3g

Edamame and Avocado Dip

Prep Time: 10 mins

Total Time: 10 mins

Servings: 4 servings

Ingredients:
- 1 cup shelled edamame, cooked
- 1 ripe avocado
- 1 garlic clove, minced
- 2 tablespoons lemon juice
- 2 tablespoons chopped fresh cilantro
- Salt and pepper to taste
- Optional: red pepper flakes for a spicy kick

Directions:
1. In a food processor or blender, combine cooked edamame, ripe avocado, minced garlic, lemon juice, chopped fresh cilantro, salt, and pepper.

2. Blend until smooth and creamy, scraping down the sides of the bowl as needed.
3. Taste and adjust seasoning as desired, adding red pepper flakes for a spicy kick if desired.
4. Transfer the dip to a serving bowl.
5. Serve with raw vegetable sticks (e.g., carrots, celery, bell peppers) or whole grain crackers for dipping.
6. Enjoy this nutritious and flavorful edamame and avocado dip as a satisfying snack option!

Nutrition Facts (per serving):
- Calories: 150
- Protein: 7g
- Fat: 9g
- Carbohydrates: 12g
- Fiber: 7g

Hummus and Veggie Wraps

Prep Time: 10 mins

Total Time: 10 mins

Servings: 2 wraps

Ingredients:
- 2 whole grain tortillas
- 1/2 cup hummus (store-bought or homemade)
- 1 cup mixed vegetables (e.g., shredded carrots, sliced cucumber, bell pepper strips)
- Handful of fresh spinach leaves

Directions:

1. Spread a generous layer of hummus onto each tortilla.
2. Arrange mixed vegetables and spinach leaves evenly over the hummus.
3. Roll up the tortillas tightly, enclosing the filling.
4. Slice each wrap in half diagonally.
5. Serve immediately, or wrap in parchment paper for a convenient on-the-go snack.

Nutrition Facts (per serving - 1 wrap):
- Calories: 200
- Protein: 7g
- Fat: 8g
- Carbohydrates: 28g
- Fiber: 6g

Banana and Almond Butter Bites

Prep Time: 5 mins

Total Time: 5 mins

Servings: 2 servings

Ingredients:
- 1 large banana, sliced
- 2 tablespoons almond butter (or peanut butter)
- Optional toppings: shredded coconut, dark chocolate chips, chopped nuts

Directions:
1. Spread almond butter onto banana slices.
2. Sprinkle with optional toppings like shredded coconut, dark chocolate chips, or chopped nuts.

3. Enjoy immediately as a delicious and nutritious snack!

Nutrition Facts (per serving):
- Calories: 180
- Protein: 4g
- Fat: 11g
- Carbohydrates: 20g
- Fiber: 3g

Greek Yogurt with Honey and Walnuts

Prep Time: 5 mins

Total Time: 5 mins

Servings: 2 servings

Ingredients:
- 1 cup plain Greek yogurt
- 2 tablespoons honey
- 1/4 cup chopped walnuts

Directions:
1. Divide Greek yogurt between two serving bowls.
2. Drizzle honey over each serving.
3. Sprinkle chopped walnuts over the top.
4. Serve immediately and enjoy this creamy and satisfying snack!

Nutrition Facts (per serving):
- Calories: 250
- Protein: 15g
- Fat: 12g
- Carbohydrates: 20g
- Fiber: 2g

Cottage Cheese with Pineapple

Prep Time: 5 mins

Total Time: 5 mins

Servings: 2 servings

Ingredients:
- 1 cup cottage cheese
- 1/2 cup diced pineapple

Directions:
1. Divide cottage cheese between two serving bowls.
2. Top each serving with diced pineapple.
3. Serve immediately or refrigerate until ready to enjoy.
4. This cottage cheese and pineapple combination provides a balance of protein and natural sweetness, making it a satisfying snack option!

Nutrition Facts (per serving):
- Calories: 150
- Protein: 14g
- Fat: 3g
- Carbohydrates: 18g
- Fiber: 2g

Roasted Edamame

Prep Time: 5 mins

Total Time: 20 mins

Servings: 2 servings

Ingredients:
- 1 cup frozen edamame, thawed

- 1 tablespoon olive oil
- 1/2 teaspoon garlic powder
- 1/2 teaspoon smoked paprika
- Salt to taste

Directions:
1. Preheat oven to 400°F (200°C). Line a baking sheet with parchment paper.
2. In a mixing bowl, toss thawed edamame with olive oil, garlic powder, smoked paprika, and salt until evenly coated.
3. Spread seasoned edamame in a single layer on the prepared baking sheet.
4. Roast in the preheated oven for 15-20 minutes, stirring halfway through, until golden brown and crispy.
5. Remove from the oven and let cool slightly before serving.
6. Enjoy these roasted edamame as a crunchy and flavorful snack option!

Nutrition Facts (per serving):
- Calories: 150
- Protein: 12g
- Fat: 7g
- Carbohydrates: 10g
- Fiber: 6g

DESSERTS RECIPES

Fruit Salad with Honey-Lime Dressing

Prep Time: 15 mins

Total Time: 15 mins

Servings: 4 servings

Ingredients:

- 2 cups mixed fruits (e.g., strawberries, blueberries, kiwi, pineapple, grapes)
- 1 tablespoon honey
- 1 tablespoon lime juice
- 1 teaspoon lime zest
- Fresh mint leaves for garnish (optional)

Directions:

1. Wash and prepare the fruits as needed, then chop them into bite-sized pieces.
2. In a small bowl, whisk together honey, lime juice, and lime zest to make the dressing.
3. Pour the dressing over the mixed fruits and toss gently to coat.
4. Garnish with fresh mint leaves if desired.
5. Serve immediately or chill in the refrigerator until ready to enjoy.

Nutrition Facts (per serving):

- Calories: 80
- Protein: 1g
- Fat: 0g

- Carbohydrates: 21g
- Fiber: 3g

Dark Chocolate Avocado Mousse

Prep Time: 10 mins

Total Time: 10 mins

Servings: 4 servings

Ingredients:
- 2 ripe avocados
- 1/4 cup unsweetened cocoa powder
- 1/4 cup honey or maple syrup
- 1 teaspoon vanilla extract
- Pinch of salt
- Fresh berries for garnish (optional)

Directions:
1. Cut the avocados in half, remove the pits, and scoop out the flesh into a food processor or blender.
2. Add cocoa powder, honey or maple syrup, vanilla extract, and a pinch of salt to the avocados.
3. Blend until smooth and creamy, scraping down the sides of the bowl as needed.
4. Divide the chocolate avocado mousse into serving dishes.
5. Chill in the refrigerator for at least 30 minutes before serving.
6. Garnish with fresh berries if desired.

Nutrition Facts (per serving):
- Calories: 200
- Protein: 3g

- Fat: 14g
- Carbohydrates: 20g
- Fiber: 7g

Baked Apples with Cinnamon

Prep Time: 10 mins

Total Time: 40 mins

Servings: 4 servings

Ingredients:

- 4 large apples
- 2 tablespoons honey or maple syrup
- 1 teaspoon ground cinnamon
- 1/4 cup chopped nuts (e.g., walnuts, pecans, almonds)

Directions:

1. Preheat the oven to 375°F (190°C). Grease a baking dish with non-stick cooking spray.
2. Wash the apples and core them using an apple corer or a knife, leaving the bottoms intact.
3. In a small bowl, mix together honey or maple syrup and ground cinnamon.
4. Place the cored apples in the prepared baking dish.
5. Fill each apple cavity with the honey-cinnamon mixture.
6. Sprinkle chopped nuts over the top of each apple.
7. Bake in the preheated oven for 30-40 minutes, or until the apples are tender.
8. Remove from the oven and let cool slightly before serving.

9. Enjoy these baked apples warm, either on their own or topped with a dollop of Greek yogurt.

Nutrition Facts (per serving):
- Calories: 150
- Protein: 2g
- Fat: 4g
- Carbohydrates: 30g
- Fiber: 5g

Chia Seed Pudding

Prep Time: 5 mins (plus chilling time)

Total Time: 4 hrs 5 mins

Servings: 4 servings

Ingredients:
- 1/2 cup chia seeds
- 2 cups unsweetened almond milk or coconut milk
- 2 tablespoons honey or maple syrup
- 1 teaspoon vanilla extract
- Fresh berries for topping (optional)

Directions:
1. In a mixing bowl, whisk together chia seeds, almond milk or coconut milk, honey or maple syrup, and vanilla extract.
2. Cover the bowl and refrigerate for at least 4 hours or overnight, allowing the chia seeds to thicken and absorb the liquid.
3. Stir the chia seed pudding well before serving.
4. Divide the pudding into serving dishes and top with fresh berries if desired.

5. Serve chilled and enjoy this creamy and nutritious dessert!

Nutrition Facts (per serving):
- Calories: 130
- Protein: 3g
- Fat: 7g
- Carbohydrates: 14g
- Fiber: 9g

Baked Banana Oatmeal Cups

Prep Time: 10 mins

Total Time: 25 mins

Servings: 12 servings

Ingredients:
- 2 ripe bananas, mashed
- 2 cups rolled oats
- 1/4 cup honey or maple syrup
- 1/4 cup unsweetened applesauce
- 1 teaspoon vanilla extract
- 1/2 teaspoon ground cinnamon
- 1/4 teaspoon salt
- Optional add-ins: chopped nuts, dried fruits, chocolate chips

Directions:
1. Preheat the oven to 350°F (175°C). Grease a muffin tin with non-stick cooking spray.
2. In a mixing bowl, combine mashed bananas, rolled oats, honey or maple syrup, applesauce, vanilla extract, ground cinnamon, salt, and any optional add-ins of your choice.

3. Divide the oatmeal mixture evenly among the prepared muffin cups.
4. Bake in the preheated oven for 15-20 minutes, or until the tops are golden brown and set.
5. Remove from the oven and let cool in the muffin tin for a few minutes before transferring to a wire rack to cool completely.
6. Once cooled, store leftover oatmeal cups in an airtight container in the refrigerator.
7. Enjoy these baked banana oatmeal cups as a wholesome and delicious dessert or snack option!

Nutrition Facts (per serving - 1 oatmeal cup):
- Calories: 120
- Protein: 3g
- Fat: 2g
- Carbohydrates: 24g
- Fiber: 3g

Blueberry Oatmeal Cookies

Prep Time: 10 mins

Total Time: 25 mins

Servings: 12 cookies

Ingredients:
- 1 cup rolled oats
- 1/2 cup almond flour
- 1/2 teaspoon baking powder
- 1/4 teaspoon salt
- 1/4 cup honey or maple syrup

- 1/4 cup unsweetened applesauce
- 1 tablespoon coconut oil, melted
- 1 teaspoon vanilla extract
- 1/2 cup fresh or frozen blueberries

Directions:
1. Preheat the oven to 350°F (175°C). Line a baking sheet with parchment paper.
2. In a mixing bowl, combine rolled oats, almond flour, baking powder, and salt.
3. In a separate bowl, whisk together honey or maple syrup, applesauce, melted coconut oil, and vanilla extract.
4. Add the wet ingredients to the dry ingredients and stir until well combined.
5. Gently fold in the blueberries.
6. Drop spoonfuls of the cookie dough onto the prepared baking sheet, spacing them apart.
7. Flatten each cookie slightly with the back of a spoon.
8. Bake in the preheated oven for 12-15 minutes, or until the edges are golden brown.
9. Remove from the oven and let the cookies cool on the baking sheet for 5 minutes before transferring them to a wire rack to cool completely.
10. Enjoy these delicious and wholesome blueberry oatmeal cookies as a guilt-free dessert or snack option!

Nutrition Facts (per serving - 1 cookie):
- Calories: 90

- Protein: 2g
- Fat: 3.5g
- Carbohydrates: 14g
- Fiber: 2g

Chia Seed Chocolate Pudding

Prep Time: 5 mins (plus chilling time)

Total Time: 4 hrs 5 mins

Servings: 4 servings

Ingredients:
- 1/4 cup chia seeds
- 1 cup unsweetened almond milk or coconut milk
- 2 tablespoons unsweetened cocoa powder
- 2 tablespoons honey or maple syrup
- 1/2 teaspoon vanilla extract
- Pinch of salt

Directions:
1. In a mixing bowl, whisk together chia seeds, almond milk or coconut milk, cocoa powder, honey or maple syrup, vanilla extract, and a pinch of salt.
2. Cover the bowl and refrigerate for at least 4 hours or overnight, allowing the chia seeds to thicken and absorb the liquid.
3. Stir the chocolate chia seed pudding well before serving.
4. Divide the pudding into serving dishes.
5. Serve chilled and enjoy this rich and creamy chocolate dessert!

Nutrition Facts (per serving):
- Calories: 100

- Protein: 3g
- Fat: 5g
- Carbohydrates: 14g
- Fiber: 6g

Baked Peach Crisp

Prep Time: 15 mins

Total Time: 45 mins

Servings: 4 servings

Ingredients:

- 4 ripe peaches, sliced
- 1 tablespoon honey or maple syrup
- 1 teaspoon lemon juice
- 1/2 teaspoon ground cinnamon
- 1/4 teaspoon ground nutmeg
- 1/2 cup rolled oats
- 1/4 cup almond flour
- 2 tablespoons coconut oil, melted
- 2 tablespoons chopped almonds or pecans

Directions:

1. Preheat the oven to 350°F (175°C). Grease a baking dish with coconut oil or non-stick cooking spray.
2. In a mixing bowl, combine sliced peaches, honey or maple syrup, lemon juice, ground cinnamon, and ground nutmeg. Toss until the peaches are evenly coated.
3. Transfer the peach mixture to the prepared baking dish, spreading it out into an even layer.

4. In a separate bowl, mix together rolled oats, almond flour, melted coconut oil, and chopped almonds or pecans until crumbly.
5. Sprinkle the oat mixture over the top of the peaches in the baking dish.
6. Bake in the preheated oven for 25-30 minutes, or until the topping is golden brown and the peaches are bubbling.
7. Remove from the oven and let cool slightly before serving.
8. Enjoy this warm and comforting baked peach crisp as a delightful dessert!

Nutrition Facts (per serving):
- Calories: 180
- Protein: 4g
- Fat: 8g
- Carbohydrates: 26g
- Fiber: 5g

Coconut Yogurt Parfait

Prep Time: 10 mins

Total Time: 10 mins

Servings: 2 servings

Ingredients:
- 1 cup unsweetened coconut yogurt
- 1/2 cup mixed berries (e.g., strawberries, blueberries, raspberries)
- 2 tablespoons unsweetened shredded coconut
- 2 tablespoons chopped nuts (e.g., almonds, walnuts)

Directions:
1. In two serving glasses or bowls, layer coconut yogurt, mixed berries, shredded coconut, and chopped nuts.
2. Repeat the layers until the glasses are filled.
3. Serve immediately and enjoy this refreshing and nutritious coconut yogurt parfait!

Nutrition Facts (per serving):
- Calories: 150
- Protein: 4g
- Fat: 9g
- Carbohydrates: 12g
- Fiber: 5g

Frozen Banana Bites

Prep Time: 10 mins
Total Time: 2 hrs 10 mins
Servings: 4 servings

Ingredients:
- 2 ripe bananas, peeled and cut into chunks
- 1/4 cup creamy almond butter or peanut butter
- 1/4 cup dark chocolate chips
- 1 tablespoon coconut oil

Directions:
1. Line a baking sheet with parchment paper.
2. Arrange banana chunks in a single layer on the prepared baking sheet.

3. In a small saucepan, melt almond butter or peanut butter with coconut oil and dark chocolate chips over low heat, stirring until smooth.
4. Drizzle the melted chocolate mixture over the banana chunks, covering them evenly.
5. Place the baking sheet in the freezer and freeze for at least 2 hours, or until the banana bites are firm.
6. Once frozen, remove from the freezer and transfer the banana bites to an airtight container for storage.
7. Enjoy these frozen banana bites straight from the freezer as a delicious and satisfying dessert or snack option!

Nutrition Facts (per serving):
- Calories: 160
- Protein: 3g
- Fat: 10g
- Carbohydrates: 18g
- Fiber: 3g

Berry Chia Seed Pudding

Prep Time: 5 mins (plus chilling time)

Total Time: 4 hrs 5 mins

Servings: 2 servings

Ingredients:
- 1/4 cup chia seeds
- 1 cup unsweetened almond milk or coconut milk
- 1 cup mixed berries (e.g., strawberries, blueberries, raspberries)
- 1 tablespoon honey or maple syrup

- 1/2 teaspoon vanilla extract
- Pinch of salt

Directions:

1. In a mixing bowl, whisk together chia seeds, almond milk or coconut milk, honey or maple syrup, vanilla extract, and a pinch of salt.
2. Cover the bowl and refrigerate for at least 4 hours or overnight, allowing the chia seeds to thicken and absorb the liquid.
3. In a blender, puree half of the mixed berries until smooth.
4. Once the chia seed pudding has set, divide it into serving glasses or bowls.
5. Pour the berry puree over the top of the pudding in each serving glass.
6. Garnish with the remaining mixed berries.
7. Serve chilled and enjoy this nutritious and flavorful berry chia seed pudding!

Nutrition Facts (per serving):

- Calories: 150
- Protein: 4g
- Fat: 6g
- Carbohydrates: 22g
- Fiber: 9g

Cinnamon Baked Apples

Prep Time: 10 mins

Total Time: 40 mins

Servings: 2 servings

Ingredients:
- 2 apples (e.g., Granny Smith, Honey crisp), cored
- 2 tablespoons chopped nuts (e.g., walnuts, almonds, pecans)
- 1 tablespoon honey or maple syrup
- 1 teaspoon ground cinnamon
- 1/4 teaspoon nutmeg (optional)
- 1 tablespoon coconut oil, melted
- 1/4 cup water

Directions:
1. Preheat the oven to 375°F (190°C). Grease a baking dish with coconut oil.
2. In a small bowl, mix together chopped nuts, honey or maple syrup, ground cinnamon, and nutmeg (if using).
3. Stuff each cored apple with the nut mixture.
4. Place the stuffed apples in the prepared baking dish.
5. Drizzle melted coconut oil over the top of the stuffed apples.
6. Pour water into the bottom of the baking dish.
7. Bake in the preheated oven for 30-35 minutes, or until the apples are tender.
8. Remove from the oven and let cool slightly before serving.
9. Enjoy these warm and comforting cinnamon baked apples as a delightful dessert!

Nutrition Facts (per serving):
- Calories: 200
- Protein: 2g
- Fat: 9g

- Carbohydrates: 31g
- Fiber: 5g

Coconut Almond Date Balls

Prep Time: 15 mins

Total Time: 15 mins

Servings: 8 balls

Ingredients:
- 1 cup pitted dates
- 1/2 cup shredded unsweetened coconut
- 1/2 cup almonds
- 1 tablespoon coconut oil, melted
- Pinch of salt

Directions:
1. In a food processor, combine pitted dates, shredded coconut, almonds, melted coconut oil, and a pinch of salt.
2. Process until the mixture forms a sticky dough.
3. Scoop out tablespoon-sized portions of the dough and roll them into balls.
4. Place the coconut almond date balls on a plate or baking sheet lined with parchment paper.
5. Refrigerate for at least 30 minutes to firm up.
6. Serve chilled and enjoy these delicious and energizing coconut almond date balls!

Nutrition Facts (per serving - 1 ball):
- Calories: 120
- Protein: 2g

- Fat: 6g
- Carbohydrates: 16g
- Fiber: 3g

Greek Yogurt with Honey and Pistachios

Prep Time: 5 mins

Total Time: 5 mins

Servings: 2 servings

Ingredients:
- 1 cup plain Greek yogurt
- 2 tablespoons honey
- 2 tablespoons chopped pistachios

Directions:
1. Divide Greek yogurt into serving bowls.
2. Drizzle honey over the top of each serving of Greek yogurt.
3. Sprinkle chopped pistachios over the yogurt and honey.
4. Serve immediately and enjoy this creamy and indulgent Greek yogurt dessert!

Nutrition Facts (per serving):
- Calories: 180
- Protein: 12g
- Fat: 6g
- Carbohydrates: 20g
- Fiber: 1g

Baked Pears with Cinnamon and Walnuts

Prep Time: 10 mins

Total Time: 30 mins

Servings: 2 servings

Ingredients:

- 2 ripe pears, halved and cored
- 2 tablespoons honey or maple syrup
- 1 teaspoon ground cinnamon
- 1/4 cup chopped walnuts

Directions:

1. Preheat the oven to 375°F (190°C). Grease a baking dish with coconut oil or non-stick cooking spray.
2. Place the pear halves, cut side up, in the prepared baking dish.
3. In a small bowl, mix together honey or maple syrup and ground cinnamon.
4. Drizzle the honey-cinnamon mixture over the top of each pear half.
5. Sprinkle chopped walnuts over the pears.
6. Bake in the preheated oven for 20-25 minutes, or until the pears are tender and caramelized.
7. Remove from the oven and let cool slightly before serving.
8. Enjoy these warm and fragrant baked pears as a delightful dessert!

Nutrition Facts (per serving):

- Calories: 200
- Protein: 2g
- Fat: 6g

- Carbohydrates: 40g
- Fiber: 6g

Almond Butter Banana Bites

Prep Time: 10 mins

Total Time: 10 mins

Servings: 2 servings

Ingredients:
- 1 ripe banana
- 2 tablespoons almond butter
- 2 tablespoons unsweetened shredded coconut
- 2 tablespoons chopped almonds or walnuts

Directions:
1. Peel the banana and slice it into rounds, about 1/2 inch thick.
2. Spread almond butter onto half of the banana slices.
3. Top each almond butter-covered banana slice with another banana slice to make a sandwich.
4. Roll the edges of the banana sandwiches in shredded coconut until coated.
5. Insert a toothpick into each banana bite to hold it together.
6. Sprinkle chopped almonds or walnuts over the top of the banana bites.
7. Serve immediately or refrigerate for a firmer texture.
8. Enjoy these delightful almond butter banana bites as a nutritious and satisfying dessert or snack!

Nutrition Facts (per serving):
- Calories: 180

- Protein: 4g
- Fat: 12g
- Carbohydrates: 17g
- Fiber: 4g

Greek Yogurt Parfait with Berries

Prep Time: 10 mins

Total Time: 10 mins

Servings: 2 servings

Ingredients:

- 1 cup plain Greek yogurt
- 1 cup mixed berries (e.g., strawberries, blueberries, raspberries)
- 2 tablespoons chopped nuts (e.g., almonds, walnuts, pecans)
- 2 tablespoons honey or maple syrup

Directions:

1. In serving glasses or bowls, layer plain Greek yogurt, mixed berries, and chopped nuts.
2. Drizzle honey or maple syrup over the top of each parfait.
3. Repeat the layers if desired.
4. Serve immediately and enjoy this simple yet delicious Greek yogurt parfait with berries!

Nutrition Facts (per serving):

- Calories: 220
- Protein: 16g
- Fat: 6g
- Carbohydrates: 28g
- Fiber: 4g

Chocolate Avocado Pudding

Prep Time: 10 mins

Total Time: 10 mins

Servings: 2 servings

Ingredients:

- 1 ripe avocado
- 2 tablespoons unsweetened cocoa powder
- 2 tablespoons honey or maple syrup
- 1/2 teaspoon vanilla extract
- Pinch of salt
- 1/4 cup unsweetened almond milk or coconut milk

Directions:

1. In a blender or food processor, combine ripe avocado, unsweetened cocoa powder, honey or maple syrup, vanilla extract, salt, and almond milk or coconut milk.
2. Blend until smooth and creamy, scraping down the sides of the blender or food processor as needed.
3. Divide the chocolate avocado pudding into serving glasses or bowls.
4. Refrigerate for at least 30 minutes to chill and set.
5. Serve chilled and enjoy this rich and indulgent chocolate avocado pudding!

Nutrition Facts (per serving):

- Calories: 200
- Protein: 3g
- Fat: 12g

- Carbohydrates: 24g
- Fiber: 7g

Fruit Salad with Mint Honey Dressing

Prep Time: 15 mins

Total Time: 15 mins

Servings: 2 servings

Ingredients:
- 1 cup mixed fresh fruit (e.g., strawberries, kiwi, pineapple, grapes)
- 1 tablespoon chopped fresh mint leaves
- 1 tablespoon honey
- 1 teaspoon lemon juice

Directions:
1. Wash and prepare the mixed fresh fruit as needed, cutting them into bite-sized pieces.
2. In a small bowl, whisk together chopped fresh mint leaves, honey, and lemon juice to make the dressing.
3. Pour the mint honey dressing over the mixed fresh fruit and gently toss to coat.
4. Divide the fruit salad into serving bowls or plates.
5. Serve immediately and enjoy this refreshing and naturally sweet fruit salad with mint honey dressing!

Nutrition Facts (per serving):
- Calories: 120
- Protein: 1g
- Fat: 0g

- Carbohydrates: 31g
- Fiber: 3g

Baked Cinnamon Apple Slices

Prep Time: 10 mins

Total Time: 30 mins

Servings: 2 servings

Ingredients:
- 2 apples (e.g., Granny Smith, Honey crisp), cored and sliced
- 1 tablespoon honey or maple syrup
- 1 teaspoon ground cinnamon
- 1 tablespoon melted coconut oil

Directions:
1. Preheat the oven to 375°F (190°C). Grease a baking dish with coconut oil.
2. In a bowl, toss the apple slices with honey or maple syrup, ground cinnamon, and melted coconut oil until evenly coated.
3. Arrange the coated apple slices in a single layer in the prepared baking dish.
4. Bake in the preheated oven for 20-25 minutes, or until the apples are tender and lightly caramelized.
5. Remove from the oven and let cool slightly before serving.
6. Enjoy these warm and aromatic baked cinnamon apple slices as a delightful dessert or snack!

Nutrition Facts (per serving):
- Calories: 140
- Protein: 1g

- Fat: 4g
- Carbohydrates: 29g
- Fiber: 5g

SEAFOOD RECIPES

Grilled Lemon Herb Salmon

Prep Time: 10 mins

Total Time: 20 mins

Servings: 2

Ingredients:

- 2 salmon fillets (6 oz each), skin-on
- 2 tablespoons olive oil
- 1 tablespoon lemon juice
- 2 cloves garlic, minced
- 1 teaspoon fresh thyme leaves
- 1 teaspoon fresh rosemary leaves
- Salt and pepper, to taste
- Lemon slices (for garnish)

Directions:

1. Preheat the grill to medium-high heat.
2. In a small bowl, whisk together olive oil, lemon juice, minced garlic, thyme, and rosemary.
3. Place the salmon fillets on a plate and brush both sides with the lemon herb marinade. Season with salt and pepper.
4. Place the salmon fillets, skin-side down, on the preheated grill. Close the lid and grill for 4-5 minutes per side, or until the salmon is cooked through and flakes easily with a fork.
5. Remove the grilled salmon from the grill and transfer to a serving platter.

6. Garnish with lemon slices and additional fresh herbs if desired.
7. Serve immediately and enjoy this flavorful grilled lemon herb salmon!

Nutrition Facts (per serving):
- Calories: 350
- Protein: 34g
- Fat: 22g
- Carbohydrates: 1g
- Fiber: 0g

Baked Lemon Garlic Shrimp

Prep Time: 10 mins

Total Time: 20 mins

Servings: 2

Ingredients:
- 1/2 lb large shrimp, peeled and deveined
- 2 tablespoons olive oil
- 2 cloves garlic, minced
- 1 tablespoon lemon juice
- 1 teaspoon lemon zest
- 1 tablespoon chopped fresh parsley
- Salt and pepper, to taste

Directions:
1. Preheat the oven to 400°F (200°C). Grease a baking dish with olive oil.

2. In a bowl, toss the shrimp with olive oil, minced garlic, lemon juice, lemon zest, chopped parsley, salt, and pepper until evenly coated.
3. Arrange the seasoned shrimp in a single layer in the prepared baking dish.
4. Bake in the preheated oven for 8-10 minutes, or until the shrimp are pink and cooked through.
5. Remove from the oven and let cool slightly before serving.
6. Serve these delicious baked lemon garlic shrimp as a flavorful and healthy seafood dish!

Nutrition Facts (per serving):
- Calories: 180
- Protein: 20g
- Fat: 10g
- Carbohydrates: 3g
- Fiber: 0g

Pan-Seared Scallops with Lemon Butter Sauce

Prep Time: 10 mins

Total Time: 10 mins

Servings: 2

Ingredients:
- 6 large scallops
- Salt and pepper, to taste
- 2 tablespoons olive oil
- 2 tablespoons unsalted butter
- 2 cloves garlic, minced

- 1 tablespoon lemon juice
- 1 tablespoon chopped fresh parsley

Directions:

1. Pat the scallops dry with paper towels and season both sides with salt and pepper.
2. Heat olive oil in a large skillet over medium-high heat.
3. Add the scallops to the skillet and cook for 2-3 minutes on each side, or until golden brown and cooked through.
4. Remove the cooked scallops from the skillet and transfer to a plate. Cover with foil to keep warm.
5. In the same skillet, melt the butter over medium heat. Add minced garlic and cook for 1 minute, or until fragrant.
6. Remove the skillet from the heat and stir in lemon juice and chopped parsley.
7. Pour the lemon butter sauce over the cooked scallops.
8. Serve immediately and enjoy these succulent pan-seared scallops with lemon butter sauce!

Nutrition Facts (per serving):

- Calories: 220
- Protein: 18g
- Fat: 15g
- Carbohydrates: 2g
- Fiber: 0g

Grilled Garlic Herb Shrimp Skewers

Prep Time: 20 mins (includes marinating time)

Total Time: 30 mins

Servings: 2

Ingredients:
- 1/2 lb large shrimp, peeled and deveined
- 2 tablespoons olive oil
- 2 cloves garlic, minced
- 1 tablespoon chopped fresh parsley
- 1 teaspoon chopped fresh thyme
- 1 teaspoon chopped fresh rosemary
- Salt and pepper, to taste
- Lemon wedges (for serving)

Directions:
1. In a bowl, combine olive oil, minced garlic, chopped parsley, thyme, rosemary, salt, and pepper.
2. Add the peeled and deveined shrimp to the marinade and toss to coat. Cover and refrigerate for at least 15 minutes.
3. Preheat the grill to medium-high heat. Thread the marinated shrimp onto skewers.
4. Grill the shrimp skewers for 2-3 minutes on each side, or until the shrimp are pink and opaque.
5. Remove from the grill and transfer the grilled shrimp skewers to a serving platter.
6. Serve with lemon wedges for squeezing over the shrimp.
7. Enjoy these flavorful grilled garlic herb shrimp skewers as a tasty and nutritious seafood dish!

Nutrition Facts (per serving):
- Calories: 190
- Protein: 20g
- Fat: 12g
- Carbohydrates: 2g
- Fiber: 0g

Baked Lemon Dijon Salmon

Prep Time: 10 mins

Total Time: 20 mins

Servings: 2

Ingredients:
- 2 salmon fillets (6 oz each)
- 2 tablespoons Dijon mustard
- 2 tablespoons olive oil
- 1 tablespoon lemon juice
- 2 cloves garlic, minced
- 1 teaspoon lemon zest
- Salt and pepper, to taste

Directions:
1. Preheat the oven to 400°F (200°C). Grease a baking dish with olive oil.
2. In a small bowl, whisk together Dijon mustard, olive oil, lemon juice, minced garlic, lemon zest, salt, and pepper.
3. Place the salmon fillets in the prepared baking dish and brush the Dijon mustard mixture over the top of each fillet.

4. Bake in the preheated oven for 12-15 minutes, or until the salmon is cooked through and flakes easily with a fork.
5. Remove from the oven and let cool slightly before serving.
6. Serve this flavorful baked lemon Dijon salmon with your favorite side dishes.
7. Enjoy this delicious and nutritious seafood dish!

Nutrition Facts (per serving):
- Calories: 320
- Protein: 34g
- Fat: 18g
- Carbohydrates: 2g
- Fiber: 0g

Lemon Garlic Shrimp Pasta

Prep Time: 10 mins

Total Time: 20 mins

Servings: 2

Ingredients:
- 8 oz whole wheat spaghetti
- 1/2 lb large shrimp, peeled and deveined
- 2 tablespoons olive oil
- 3 cloves garlic, minced
- 1 tablespoon lemon juice
- 1 teaspoon lemon zest
- Salt and pepper, to taste
- 2 tablespoons chopped fresh parsley
- Grated Parmesan cheese (optional, for serving)

Directions:

1. Cook the spaghetti according to package instructions until al dente. Drain and set aside.
2. In a large skillet, heat olive oil over medium heat. Add minced garlic and cook for 1 minute, or until fragrant.
3. Add the shrimp to the skillet and cook for 2-3 minutes on each side, or until pink and cooked through.
4. Stir in lemon juice, lemon zest, salt, pepper, and chopped parsley.
5. Add the cooked spaghetti to the skillet and toss to coat with the shrimp and lemon garlic sauce.
6. Cook for an additional 1-2 minutes, stirring occasionally, until heated through.
7. Serve the lemon garlic shrimp pasta hot, garnished with grated Parmesan cheese if desired.

Nutritional Information (per serving):

- Calories: 430
- Protein: 26g
- Fat: 14g
- Carbohydrates: 53g
- Fiber: 6g

Grilled Salmon with Avocado Salsa

Prep Time: 10 mins

Total Time: 20 mins

Servings: 2

Ingredients:

- 2 salmon fillets (6 oz each)
- 1 tablespoon olive oil
- Salt and pepper, to taste
- 1 avocado, diced
- 1 tomato, diced
- 1/4 red onion, finely chopped
- 1 tablespoon chopped fresh cilantro
- 1 tablespoon lime juice

Directions:
1. Preheat the grill to medium-high heat. Brush the salmon fillets with olive oil and season with salt and pepper.
2. Grill the salmon fillets for 4-5 minutes on each side, or until cooked through and flaky.
3. In a bowl, combine diced avocado, tomato, red onion, cilantro, and lime juice to make the avocado salsa.
4. Serve the grilled salmon topped with avocado salsa.

Nutritional Information (per serving):
- Calories: 380
- Protein: 26g
- Fat: 25g
- Carbohydrates: 12g
- Fiber: 6g

Shrimp and Vegetable Stir-Fry

Prep Time: 15 mins

Total Time: 20 mins

Servings: 2

Ingredients:
- 1/2 lb large shrimp, peeled and deveined
- 2 tablespoons olive oil
- 2 cloves garlic, minced
- 1 bell pepper, thinly sliced
- 1 cup broccoli florets
- 1 carrot, thinly sliced
- 1/4 cup low-sodium soy sauce
- 1 tablespoon honey
- 1 teaspoon sesame oil
- 1 tablespoon cornstarch
- Cooked brown rice, for serving

Directions:
1. In a small bowl, whisk together soy sauce, honey, sesame oil, and cornstarch to make the sauce. Set aside.
2. Heat olive oil in a large skillet or wok over medium-high heat. Add minced garlic and cook for 1 minute.
3. Add shrimp to the skillet and cook for 2-3 minutes on each side, or until pink and cooked through. Remove shrimp from the skillet and set aside.
4. In the same skillet, add bell pepper, broccoli, and carrot. Stir-fry for 3-4 minutes, or until vegetables are tender-crisp.
5. Return the cooked shrimp to the skillet and pour the sauce over the shrimp and vegetables. Cook for an additional 1-2 minutes, stirring constantly, until the sauce thickens.

6. Serve the shrimp and vegetable stir-fry hot over cooked brown rice.

Nutritional Information (per serving):
- Calories: 350
- Protein: 25g
- Fat: 14g
- Carbohydrates: 30g
- Fiber: 5g

Tuna Salad Stuffed Avocados

Prep Time: 10 mins

Total Time: 10 mins

Servings: 2

Ingredients:
- 1 can (5 oz) tuna, drained
- 2 ripe avocados
- 1/4 cup diced cucumber
- 1/4 cup diced red bell pepper
- 2 tablespoons chopped fresh parsley
- 1 tablespoon lemon juice
- Salt and pepper, to taste

Directions:
1. Cut the avocados in half and remove the pits. Scoop out some of the flesh from each avocado half to create a larger cavity for the filling.

2. In a bowl, combine drained tuna, diced cucumber, diced red bell pepper, chopped parsley, lemon juice, salt, and pepper. Mix until well combined.
3. Spoon the tuna salad mixture into the avocado halves, dividing evenly.
4. Serve the tuna salad stuffed avocados immediately as a delicious and nutritious seafood snack or light meal.

Nutritional Information (per serving):
- Calories: 280
- Protein: 18g
- Fat: 20g
- Carbohydrates: 12g
- Fiber: 9g

Baked Cod with Lemon Herb Crust

Prep Time: 10 mins
Total Time: 20 mins
Servings: 2

Ingredients:
- 2 cod fillets (6 oz each)
- 1 tablespoon olive oil
- 1 tablespoon lemon juice
- 1 teaspoon lemon zest
- 1 tablespoon chopped fresh parsley
- 1 tablespoon chopped fresh dill
- Salt and pepper, to taste
- Lemon wedges (for serving)

Directions:
1. Preheat the oven to 400°F (200°C). Grease a baking dish with olive oil.
2. In a small bowl, combine olive oil, lemon juice, lemon zest, chopped parsley, chopped dill, salt, and pepper.
3. Place the cod fillets in the prepared baking dish and brush both sides with the lemon herb mixture.
4. Bake in the preheated oven for 12-15 minutes, or until the cod is opaque and flakes easily with a fork.
5. Remove from the oven and serve the baked cod hot, garnished with lemon wedges.

Nutritional Information (per serving):
- Calories: 260
- Protein: 26g
- Fat: 10g
- Carbohydrates: 2g
- Fiber: 1g

Herb-Crusted Baked Salmon

Prep Time: 10 mins

Total Time: 25 mins

Servings: 2

Ingredients:
- 2 salmon fillets (6 oz each)
- 2 tablespoons whole wheat breadcrumbs
- 1 tablespoon chopped fresh parsley
- 1 tablespoon chopped fresh dill

- 1 tablespoon olive oil
- 1 tablespoon Dijon mustard
- Salt and pepper, to taste
- Lemon wedges (for serving)

Directions:
1. Preheat the oven to 400°F (200°C). Line a baking sheet with parchment paper.
2. In a small bowl, combine breadcrumbs, chopped parsley, chopped dill, olive oil, Dijon mustard, salt, and pepper to form the herb crust.
3. Place the salmon fillets on the prepared baking sheet. Spread the herb crust mixture evenly over the top of each fillet, pressing gently to adhere.
4. Bake in the preheated oven for 12-15 minutes, or until the salmon is cooked through and flakes easily with a fork.
5. Remove from the oven and serve the herb-crusted baked salmon hot, garnished with lemon wedges.

Nutritional Information (per serving):
- Calories: 320
- Protein: 26g
- Fat: 20g
- Carbohydrates: 4g
- Fiber: 1g

Coconut Shrimp with Mango Salsa

Prep Time: 15 mins

Total Time: 20 mins

Servings: 2

Ingredients:

- 1/2 lb large shrimp, peeled and deveined
- 1/2 cup unsweetened shredded coconut
- 1 egg, beaten
- 1/4 cup whole wheat flour
- 1/2 teaspoon paprika
- Salt and pepper, to taste
- 1 mango, diced
- 1/4 cup diced red bell pepper
- 1/4 cup chopped fresh cilantro
- 1 tablespoon lime juice

Directions:

1. Preheat the oven to 400°F (200°C). Line a baking sheet with parchment paper.
2. In separate bowls, place beaten egg, whole wheat flour mixed with paprika, and shredded coconut.
3. Dip each shrimp into the flour mixture, then into the beaten egg, and finally into the shredded coconut, pressing gently to coat.
4. Place the coated shrimp on the prepared baking sheet. Season with salt and pepper.
5. Bake in the preheated oven for 10-12 minutes, or until the coconut coating is golden brown and the shrimp are cooked through.

6. In the meantime, prepare the mango salsa by combining diced mango, diced red bell pepper, chopped cilantro, and lime juice in a bowl.
7. Serve the coconut shrimp hot with mango salsa on the side.

Nutritional Information (per serving):
- Calories: 290
- Protein: 20g
- Fat: 12g
- Carbohydrates: 25g
- Fiber: 5g

Tilapia Piccata

Prep Time: 10 mins

Total Time: 20 mins

Servings: 2

Ingredients:
- 2 tilapia fillets (6 oz each)
- 2 tablespoons whole wheat flour
- 2 tablespoons olive oil
- 2 tablespoons lemon juice
- 1/4 cup low-sodium chicken broth
- 2 tablespoons capers, drained
- 2 tablespoons chopped fresh parsley
- Salt and pepper, to taste

Directions:
1. Season the tilapia fillets with salt and pepper, then dredge them in whole wheat flour, shaking off any excess.

2. Heat olive oil in a large skillet over medium-high heat. Add the tilapia fillets and cook for 3-4 minutes on each side, or until golden brown and cooked through. Remove from skillet and set aside.
3. In the same skillet, add lemon juice, chicken broth, and capers. Bring to a simmer and cook for 2 minutes, stirring occasionally.
4. Return the cooked tilapia fillets to the skillet, spooning the sauce over the top.
5. Cook for an additional 1-2 minutes, until the fish is heated through.
6. Serve the tilapia piccata hot, garnished with chopped fresh parsley.

Nutritional Information (per serving):
- Calories: 280
- Protein: 30g
- Fat: 14g
- Carbohydrates: 8g
- Fiber: 1g

Grilled Halibut with Lemon Herb Sauce

Prep Time: 15 mins

Total Time: 20 mins

Servings: 2

Ingredients:
- 2 halibut fillets (6 oz each)
- 1 tablespoon olive oil
- 1 tablespoon lemon juice

- 1 teaspoon lemon zest
- 1 tablespoon chopped fresh parsley
- 1 tablespoon chopped fresh dill
- Salt and pepper, to taste

Directions:

1. Preheat the grill to medium-high heat. Brush halibut fillets with olive oil and season with salt and pepper.
2. In a small bowl, combine lemon juice, lemon zest, chopped parsley, and chopped dill to make the lemon herb sauce.
3. Grill the halibut fillets for 3-4 minutes on each side, or until cooked through and opaque.
4. Remove the grilled halibut from the grill and drizzle with the lemon herb sauce.
5. Serve the grilled halibut hot, garnished with additional chopped fresh parsley and dill if desired.

Nutritional Information (per serving):

- Calories: 290
- Protein: 28g
- Fat: 12g
- Carbohydrates: 2g
- Fiber: 1g

Lemon Garlic Shrimp with Quinoa

Prep Time: 10 mins

Total Time: 20 mins

Servings: 2

Ingredients:

- 1 cup quinoa, rinsed
- 1 lb large shrimp, peeled and deveined
- 2 tablespoons olive oil
- 3 cloves garlic, minced
- Zest and juice of 1 lemon
- Salt and pepper, to taste
- Chopped fresh parsley, for garnish

Directions:

1. In a medium saucepan, bring 2 cups of water to a boil. Add the quinoa, reduce heat to low, cover, and simmer for 15 minutes, or until quinoa is tender and water is absorbed.
2. In a large skillet, heat olive oil over medium-high heat. Add minced garlic and cook for 1 minute, or until fragrant.
3. Add the shrimp to the skillet and cook for 2-3 minutes on each side, or until pink and cooked through.
4. Stir in lemon zest and lemon juice. Season with salt and pepper to taste.
5. Serve the lemon garlic shrimp over cooked quinoa, garnished with chopped fresh parsley.

Nutritional Information (per serving):

- Calories: 430
- Protein: 36g
- Fat: 14g
- Carbohydrates: 39g
- Fiber: 4g

Baked Cod with Tomato Basil Relish

Prep Time: 15 mins

Total Time: 25 mins

Servings: 2

Ingredients:

- 2 cod fillets (6 oz each)
- 1 cup cherry tomatoes, halved
- 2 tablespoons chopped fresh basil
- 1 tablespoon olive oil
- 1 tablespoon balsamic vinegar
- Salt and pepper, to taste

Directions:

1. Preheat the oven to 400°F (200°C). Line a baking sheet with parchment paper.
2. Place the cod fillets on the prepared baking sheet. Season with salt and pepper.
3. In a small bowl, combine cherry tomatoes, chopped basil, olive oil, and balsamic vinegar to make the tomato basil relish.
4. Spoon the tomato basil relish over the top of each cod fillet.
5. Bake in the preheated oven for 12-15 minutes, or until the cod is cooked through and flakes easily with a fork.
6. Serve the baked cod hot, topped with additional tomato basil relish if desired.

Nutritional Information (per serving):

- Calories: 270
- Protein: 32g
- Fat: 10g

- Carbohydrates: 10g
- Fiber: 2g

Cajun Grilled Shrimp Skewers

Prep Time: 15 mins

Total Time: 20 mins

Servings: 2

Ingredients:

- 1 lb large shrimp, peeled and deveined
- 2 tablespoons olive oil
- 1 tablespoon Cajun seasoning
- 1 tablespoon lemon juice
- Salt and pepper, to taste
- Lemon wedges, for serving

Directions:

1. Preheat the grill to medium-high heat.
2. In a bowl, toss the shrimp with olive oil, Cajun seasoning, lemon juice, salt, and pepper until evenly coated.
3. Thread the seasoned shrimp onto skewers.
4. Grill the shrimp skewers for 2-3 minutes on each side, or until pink and cooked through.
5. Remove from the grill and serve the Cajun grilled shrimp skewers hot, with lemon wedges on the side.

Nutritional Information (per serving):

- Calories: 240
- Protein: 30g
- Fat: 12g

- Carbohydrates: 2g
- Fiber: 0g

Salmon Cakes with Avocado Yogurt Sauce

Prep Time: 15 mins

Total Time: 25 mins

Servings: 2

Ingredients:

- 1 can (6 oz) wild-caught salmon, drained and flaked
- 1/4 cup whole wheat breadcrumbs
- 1 egg, beaten
- 2 tablespoons chopped fresh parsley
- 1 tablespoon chopped fresh dill
- 1/4 teaspoon garlic powder
- Salt and pepper, to taste
- 1 tablespoon olive oil
- 1 avocado, mashed
- 1/4 cup plain Greek yogurt
- 1 tablespoon lemon juice

Directions:

1. In a bowl, combine flaked salmon, breadcrumbs, beaten egg, chopped parsley, chopped dill, garlic powder, salt, and pepper. Mix until well combined.
2. Form the salmon mixture into patties.
3. Heat olive oil in a skillet over medium heat. Cook salmon cakes for 3-4 minutes on each side, or until golden brown and heated through.

4. In a small bowl, mix mashed avocado, Greek yogurt, and lemon juice to make the avocado yogurt sauce.
5. Serve the salmon cakes hot, topped with avocado yogurt sauce.

Nutritional Information (per serving):
- Calories: 320
- Protein: 25g
- Fat: 20g
- Carbohydrates: 15g
- Fiber: 6g

SOUP RECIPES

Creamy Butternut Squash Soup

Prep Time: 15 mins

Total Time: 45 mins

Servings: 4

Ingredients:

- 1 medium butternut squash, peeled, seeded, and diced
- 1 tablespoon olive oil
- 1 onion, chopped
- 2 cloves garlic, minced
- 4 cups vegetable broth
- 1 teaspoon dried thyme
- 1/2 teaspoon ground nutmeg
- Salt and pepper, to taste
- 1/2 cup coconut milk
- Fresh parsley, for garnish (optional)

Directions:

1. In a large pot, heat olive oil over medium heat. Add chopped onion and minced garlic, and cook until softened, about 5 minutes.
2. Add diced butternut squash to the pot along with vegetable broth, dried thyme, ground nutmeg, salt, and pepper. Bring to a boil, then reduce heat to low and simmer for 25-30 minutes, or until squash is tender.

3. Use an immersion blender to puree the soup until smooth. Alternatively, carefully transfer the soup to a blender and blend until smooth, then return to the pot.
4. Stir in coconut milk and cook for an additional 5 minutes, until heated through.
5. Serve the creamy butternut squash soup hot, garnished with fresh parsley if desired.

Nutritional Information (per serving):
- Calories: 170
- Protein: 3g
- Fat: 8g
- Carbohydrates: 25g
- Fiber: 6g

Lentil and Vegetable Soup

Prep Time: 15 mins

Total Time: 45 mins

Servings: 4

Ingredients:
- 1 cup dried green lentils, rinsed
- 1 tablespoon olive oil
- 1 onion, chopped
- 2 carrots, diced
- 2 celery stalks, diced
- 2 cloves garlic, minced
- 6 cups vegetable broth
- 1 can (14 oz) diced tomatoes

- 1 teaspoon ground cumin
- 1 teaspoon paprika
- Salt and pepper, to taste
- Fresh parsley, for garnish (optional)

Directions:

1. In a large pot, heat olive oil over medium heat. Add chopped onion, diced carrots, diced celery, and minced garlic. Cook until vegetables are softened, about 5 minutes.
2. Add rinsed lentils, vegetable broth, diced tomatoes, ground cumin, paprika, salt, and pepper to the pot. Bring to a boil, then reduce heat to low and simmer for 25-30 minutes, or until lentils are tender.
3. Taste and adjust seasoning if necessary.
4. Serve the lentil and vegetable soup hot, garnished with fresh parsley if desired.

Nutritional Information (per serving):

- Calories: 250
- Protein: 15g
- Fat: 4g
- Carbohydrates: 40g
- Fiber: 15g

Coconut Curry Shrimp Soup

Prep Time: 15 mins

Total Time: 30 mins

Servings: 4

Ingredients:

- 1 lb shrimp, peeled and deveined
- 1 tablespoon olive oil
- 1 onion, chopped
- 2 cloves garlic, minced
- 1 tablespoon curry powder
- 1 can (14 oz) coconut milk
- 4 cups vegetable broth
- 1 bell pepper, diced
- 1 cup sliced mushrooms
- 2 cups baby spinach
- Salt and pepper, to taste
- Fresh cilantro, for garnish (optional)

Directions:

1. In a large pot, heat olive oil over medium heat. Add chopped onion and minced garlic, and cook until softened, about 5 minutes.
2. Stir in curry powder and cook for 1 minute, until fragrant.
3. Add coconut milk and vegetable broth to the pot, and bring to a simmer.
4. Add diced bell pepper and sliced mushrooms, and simmer for 5 minutes.
5. Add shrimp and baby spinach to the pot, and cook for an additional 3-4 minutes, or until shrimp is pink and cooked through.
6. Season with salt and pepper to taste.

7. Serve the coconut curry shrimp soup hot, garnished with fresh cilantro if desired.

Nutritional Information (per serving):
- Calories: 290
- Protein: 20g
- Fat: 20g
- Carbohydrates: 10g
- Fiber: 3g

Tomato Basil Soup

Prep Time: 10 mins

Total Time: 35 mins

Servings: 4

Ingredients:
- 2 tablespoons olive oil
- 1 onion, chopped
- 2 cloves garlic, minced
- 1 can (28 oz) crushed tomatoes
- 4 cups vegetable broth
- 1/4 cup chopped fresh basil
- Salt and pepper, to taste
- 1/4 cup plain Greek yogurt, for serving (optional)

Directions:
1. In a large pot, heat olive oil over medium heat. Add chopped onion and minced garlic, and cook until softened, about 5 minutes.

2. Add crushed tomatoes and vegetable broth to the pot, and bring to a simmer.
3. Simmer the soup for 20 minutes, stirring occasionally.
4. Stir in chopped fresh basil, and season with salt and pepper to taste.
5. Use an immersion blender to puree the soup until smooth. Alternatively, carefully transfer the soup to a blender and blend until smooth, then return to the pot.
6. Serve the tomato basil soup hot, with a dollop of plain Greek yogurt on top if desired.

Nutritional Information (per serving):
- Calories: 140
- Protein: 4g
- Fat: 7g
- Carbohydrates: 17g
- Fiber: 4g

Miso Soup with Tofu and Seaweed

Prep Time: 10 mins

Total Time: 20 mins

Servings: 4

Ingredients:
- 4 cups vegetable broth
- 2 tablespoons white miso paste
- 1 block (12 oz) firm tofu, diced
- 2 green onions, thinly sliced
- 1 sheet nori seaweed, torn into small pieces

- 1 tablespoon soy sauce
- 1 teaspoon sesame oil
- 1 teaspoon rice vinegar
- 1 teaspoon grated fresh ginger

Directions:

1. In a large pot, bring vegetable broth to a simmer over medium heat.
2. In a small bowl, whisk together white miso paste and a ladleful of hot broth until smooth. Stir the miso mixture back into the pot.
3. Add diced tofu, sliced green onions, torn nori seaweed, soy sauce, sesame oil, rice vinegar, and grated fresh ginger to the pot. Simmer for 5 minutes.
4. Taste and adjust seasoning if necessary.
5. Serve the miso soup hot.

Nutritional Information (per serving):

- Calories: 150
- Protein: 11g
- Fat: 8g
- Carbohydrates: 10g
- Fiber: 2g

Creamy Spinach and Chickpea Soup

Prep Time: 10 mins

Total Time: 30 mins

Servings: 4

Ingredients:

- 1 tablespoon olive oil
- 1 onion, chopped
- 2 cloves garlic, minced
- 4 cups vegetable broth
- 2 cups chopped spinach
- 1 can (15 oz) chickpeas, drained and rinsed
- 1/2 teaspoon ground cumin
- 1/2 teaspoon ground coriander
- Salt and pepper, to taste
- 1/4 cup plain Greek yogurt, for serving (optional)
- Fresh cilantro, for garnish (optional)

Directions:

1. Heat olive oil in a large pot over medium heat. Add chopped onion and minced garlic, and cook until softened, about 5 minutes.
2. Pour vegetable broth into the pot and bring to a simmer.
3. Add chopped spinach, chickpeas, ground cumin, and ground coriander to the pot. Simmer for 15 minutes.
4. Use an immersion blender to blend the soup until smooth. Alternatively, carefully transfer the soup to a blender and blend until smooth, then return to the pot.
5. Season with salt and pepper to taste.
6. Serve the creamy spinach and chickpea soup hot, with a dollop of plain Greek yogurt on top and garnished with fresh cilantro if desired.

Nutritional Information (per serving):

- Calories: 180
- Protein: 9g
- Fat: 5g
- Carbohydrates: 26g
- Fiber: 6g

Vegetable Quinoa Soup

Prep Time: 15 mins

Total Time: 40 mins

Servings: 4

Ingredients:

- 1 tablespoon olive oil
- 1 onion, chopped
- 2 cloves garlic, minced
- 4 cups vegetable broth
- 1 can (14 oz) diced tomatoes
- 1 cup cooked quinoa
- 2 carrots, diced
- 2 celery stalks, diced
- 1 zucchini, diced
- 1 teaspoon dried thyme
- Salt and pepper, to taste
- Fresh parsley, for garnish (optional)

Directions:

1. Heat olive oil in a large pot over medium heat. Add chopped onion and minced garlic, and cook until softened, about 5 minutes.

2. Pour vegetable broth into the pot and bring to a simmer.
3. Add diced tomatoes, cooked quinoa, diced carrots, diced celery, diced zucchini, dried thyme, salt, and pepper to the pot. Simmer for 20 minutes.
4. Taste and adjust seasoning if necessary.
5. Serve the vegetable quinoa soup hot, garnished with fresh parsley if desired.

Nutritional Information (per serving):
- Calories: 220
- Protein: 7g
- Fat: 5g
- Carbohydrates: 38g
- Fiber: 7g

Ginger Carrot Soup

Prep Time: 10 mins

Total Time: 30 mins

Servings: 4

Ingredients:
- 1 tablespoon olive oil
- 1 onion, chopped
- 2 cloves garlic, minced
- 1 tablespoon fresh ginger, grated
- 6 cups vegetable broth
- 1 lb carrots, peeled and chopped
- 1 potato, peeled and chopped
- Salt and pepper, to taste

- 2 tablespoons fresh lemon juice
- Fresh cilantro, for garnish (optional)

Directions:
1. Heat olive oil in a large pot over medium heat. Add chopped onion, minced garlic, and grated ginger, and cook until softened, about 5 minutes.
2. Pour vegetable broth into the pot and bring to a simmer.
3. Add chopped carrots and chopped potato to the pot. Simmer for 15-20 minutes, or until vegetables are tender.
4. Use an immersion blender to blend the soup until smooth. Alternatively, carefully transfer the soup to a blender and blend until smooth, then return to the pot.
5. Season with salt, pepper, and fresh lemon juice to taste.
6. Serve the ginger carrot soup hot, garnished with fresh cilantro if desired.

Nutritional Information (per serving):
- Calories: 140
- Protein: 3g
- Fat: 4g
- Carbohydrates: 24g
- Fiber: 5g

Creamy Mushroom Soup

Prep Time: 10 mins
Total Time: 35 mins
Servings: 4

Ingredients:

- 1 tablespoon olive oil
- 1 onion, chopped
- 2 cloves garlic, minced
- 8 oz mushrooms, sliced
- 4 cups vegetable broth
- 1 tablespoon soy sauce
- 1 tablespoon nutritional yeast
- Salt and pepper, to taste
- 1/4 cup plain Greek yogurt, for serving (optional)
- Fresh parsley, for garnish (optional)

Directions:

1. Heat olive oil in a large pot over medium heat. Add chopped onion and minced garlic, and cook until softened, about 5 minutes.
2. Add sliced mushrooms to the pot and cook until they release their moisture and start to brown, about 8 minutes.
3. Pour vegetable broth into the pot and bring to a simmer.
4. Stir in soy sauce and nutritional yeast. Simmer for 10 minutes.
5. Use an immersion blender to blend the soup until smooth. Alternatively, carefully transfer the soup to a blender and blend until smooth, then return to the pot.
6. Season with salt and pepper to taste.
7. Serve the creamy mushroom soup hot, with a dollop of plain Greek yogurt on top and garnished with fresh parsley if desired.

Nutritional Information (per serving):

- Calories: 120

- Protein: 6g
- Fat: 4g
- Carbohydrates: 16g
- Fiber: 3g

Lentil Vegetable Soup

Prep Time: 15 mins

Total Time: 40 mins

Servings: 4

Ingredients:

- 1 tablespoon olive oil
- 1 onion, chopped
- 2 cloves garlic, minced
- 1 carrot, diced
- 1 celery stalk, diced
- 1 cup dry green lentils, rinsed
- 4 cups vegetable broth
- 1 can (14 oz) diced tomatoes
- 1 teaspoon ground cumin
- 1 teaspoon ground coriander
- Salt and pepper, to taste
- Fresh parsley, for garnish (optional)

Directions:

1. Heat olive oil in a large pot over medium heat. Add chopped onion and minced garlic, and cook until softened, about 5 minutes.

2. Add diced carrot and diced celery to the pot, and cook for another 5 minutes.
3. Stir in dry green lentils, vegetable broth, diced tomatoes, ground cumin, and ground coriander. Bring to a simmer and cook for 25-30 minutes, or until lentils are tender.
4. Taste and adjust seasoning if necessary.
5. Serve the lentil vegetable soup hot, garnished with fresh parsley if desired.

Nutritional Information (per serving):
- Calories: 240
- Protein: 13g
- Fat: 3g
- Carbohydrates: 42g
- Fiber: 15g

Detox Lentil Soup

Prep Time: 15 mins

Total Time: 45 mins

Servings: 4

Ingredients:
- 1 tablespoon olive oil
- 1 onion, chopped
- 2 cloves garlic, minced
- 2 carrots, diced
- 2 celery stalks, diced
- 1 cup dry green lentils, rinsed
- 4 cups vegetable broth

- 1 teaspoon ground cumin
- 1 teaspoon ground turmeric
- Salt and pepper, to taste
- Fresh parsley, for garnish (optional)
- Lemon wedges, for serving (optional)

Directions:

1. Heat olive oil in a large pot over medium heat. Add chopped onion and minced garlic, and cook until softened, about 5 minutes.
2. Add diced carrots and diced celery to the pot, and cook for another 5 minutes.
3. Stir in dry green lentils, vegetable broth, ground cumin, and ground turmeric. Bring to a simmer and cook for 25-30 minutes, or until lentils are tender.
4. Taste and adjust seasoning if necessary.
5. Serve the detox lentil soup hot, garnished with fresh parsley and lemon wedges if desired.

Nutritional Information (per serving):

- Calories: 220
- Protein: 12g
- Fat: 4g
- Carbohydrates: 36g
- Fiber: 15g

Creamy Cauliflower Soup

Prep Time: 10 mins

Total Time: 30 mins

Servings: 4

Ingredients:

- 1 tablespoon olive oil
- 1 onion, chopped
- 2 cloves garlic, minced
- 1 head cauliflower, chopped
- 4 cups vegetable broth
- 1 cup unsweetened almond milk
- Salt and pepper, to taste
- Fresh chives, for garnish (optional)

Directions:

1. Heat olive oil in a large pot over medium heat. Add chopped onion and minced garlic, and cook until softened, about 5 minutes.
2. Add chopped cauliflower to the pot and cook for another 5 minutes.
3. Pour vegetable broth into the pot and bring to a simmer. Cook until cauliflower is tender, about 15-20 minutes.
4. Use an immersion blender to blend the soup until smooth. Alternatively, carefully transfer the soup to a blender and blend until smooth, then return to the pot.
5. Stir in unsweetened almond milk and season with salt and pepper to taste.
6. Serve the creamy cauliflower soup hot, garnished with fresh chives if desired.

Nutritional Information (per serving):

- Calories: 120
- Protein: 3g
- Fat: 5g
- Carbohydrates: 15g
- Fiber: 5g

Tomato Basil Soup

Prep Time: 10 mins

Total Time: 30 mins

Servings: 4

Ingredients:

- 1 tablespoon olive oil
- 1 onion, chopped
- 2 cloves garlic, minced
- 2 cans (14 oz each) diced tomatoes
- 2 cups vegetable broth
- 1/4 cup fresh basil leaves, chopped
- Salt and pepper, to taste
- 1/4 cup plain Greek yogurt, for serving (optional)
- Fresh basil leaves, for garnish (optional)

Directions:

1. Heat olive oil in a large pot over medium heat. Add chopped onion and minced garlic, and cook until softened, about 5 minutes.
2. Add diced tomatoes (with their juices) and vegetable broth to the pot. Bring to a simmer and cook for 15 minutes.

3. Stir in chopped basil leaves and season with salt and pepper to taste.
4. Use an immersion blender to blend the soup until smooth. Alternatively, carefully transfer the soup to a blender and blend until smooth, then return to the pot.
5. Serve the tomato basil soup hot, with a dollop of plain Greek yogurt on top and garnished with fresh basil leaves if desired.

Nutritional Information (per serving):
- Calories: 100
- Protein: 3g
- Fat: 3g
- Carbohydrates: 16g
- Fiber: 5g

Coconut Curry Lentil Soup

Prep Time: 15 mins

Total Time: 45 mins

Servings: 4

Ingredients:
- 1 tablespoon olive oil
- 1 onion, chopped
- 2 cloves garlic, minced
- 2 carrots, diced
- 2 celery stalks, diced
- 1 cup dry red lentils, rinsed
- 4 cups vegetable broth
- 1 can (14 oz) coconut milk

- 2 tablespoons curry powder
- Salt and pepper, to taste
- Fresh cilantro, for garnish (optional)

Directions:

1. Heat olive oil in a large pot over medium heat. Add chopped onion and minced garlic, and cook until softened, about 5 minutes.
2. Add diced carrots and diced celery to the pot, and cook for another 5 minutes.
3. Stir in dry red lentils, vegetable broth, coconut milk, and curry powder. Bring to a simmer and cook for 25-30 minutes, or until lentils are tender.
4. Taste and adjust seasoning if necessary.
5. Serve the coconut curry lentil soup hot, garnished with fresh cilantro if desired.

Nutritional Information (per serving):

- Calories: 320
- Protein: 13g
- Fat: 18g
- Carbohydrates: 31g
- Fiber: 15g

Miso Mushroom Soup

Prep Time: 10 mins
Total Time: 25 mins
Servings: 4

Ingredients:

- 4 cups vegetable broth
- 2 cups water
- 4 ounces' shiitake mushrooms, sliced
- 4 ounces' button mushrooms, sliced
- 2 tablespoons miso paste
- 2 green onions, thinly sliced
- 1 tablespoon soy sauce
- 1 teaspoon sesame oil
- 1 teaspoon grated ginger
- 2 cloves garlic, minced
- Fresh cilantro, for garnish (optional)
- Red pepper flakes, for garnish (optional)

Directions:
1. In a large pot, bring vegetable broth and water to a simmer over medium heat.
2. Add sliced shiitake mushrooms and button mushrooms to the pot, and simmer for 10 minutes.
3. In a small bowl, whisk together miso paste and a ladleful of hot broth until smooth. Stir the miso mixture back into the pot.
4. Add thinly sliced green onions, soy sauce, sesame oil, grated ginger, and minced garlic to the pot. Simmer for an additional 5 minutes.
5. Taste and adjust seasoning if necessary.
6. Serve the miso mushroom soup hot, garnished with fresh cilantro and red pepper flakes if desired.

Nutritional Information (per serving):

- Calories: 70
- Protein: 4g
- Fat: 2g
- Carbohydrates: 10g
- Fiber: 2g

Detox Lentil Soup

Prep Time: 15 mins
Total Time: 45 mins
Servings: 4

Ingredients:

- 1 tablespoon olive oil
- 1 onion, chopped
- 2 cloves garlic, minced
- 2 carrots, diced
- 2 celery stalks, diced
- 1 cup dry green lentils, rinsed
- 4 cups vegetable broth
- 1 teaspoon ground cumin
- 1 teaspoon ground turmeric
- Salt and pepper, to taste
- Fresh parsley, for garnish (optional)
- Lemon wedges, for serving (optional)

Directions:

1. Heat olive oil in a large pot over medium heat. Add chopped onion and minced garlic, and cook until softened, about 5 minutes.

2. Add diced carrots and diced celery to the pot, and cook for another 5 minutes.
3. Stir in dry green lentils, vegetable broth, ground cumin, and ground turmeric. Bring to a simmer and cook for 25-30 minutes, or until lentils are tender.
4. Taste and adjust seasoning if necessary.
5. Serve the detox lentil soup hot, garnished with fresh parsley and lemon wedges if desired.

Nutritional Information (per serving):
- Calories: 220
- Protein: 12g
- Fat: 4g
- Carbohydrates: 36g
- Fiber: 15g

Creamy Cauliflower Soup

Prep Time: 10 mins

Total Time: 30 mins

Servings: 4

Ingredients:
- 1 tablespoon olive oil
- 1 onion, chopped
- 2 cloves garlic, minced
- 1 head cauliflower, chopped
- 4 cups vegetable broth
- 1 cup unsweetened almond milk
- Salt and pepper, to taste

- Fresh chives, for garnish (optional)

Directions:
1. Heat olive oil in a large pot over medium heat. Add chopped onion and minced garlic, and cook until softened, about 5 minutes.
2. Add chopped cauliflower to the pot and cook for another 5 minutes.
3. Pour vegetable broth into the pot and bring to a simmer. Cook until cauliflower is tender, about 15-20 minutes.
4. Use an immersion blender to blend the soup until smooth. Alternatively, carefully transfer the soup to a blender and blend until smooth, then return to the pot.
5. Stir in unsweetened almond milk and season with salt and pepper to taste.
6. Serve the creamy cauliflower soup hot, garnished with fresh chives if desired.

Nutritional Information (per serving):
- Calories: 120
- Protein: 3g
- Fat: 5g
- Carbohydrates: 15g
- Fiber: 5g

Tomato Basil Soup

Prep Time: 10 mins
Total Time: 30 mins
Servings: 4

Ingredients:
- 1 tablespoon olive oil
- 1 onion, chopped
- 2 cloves garlic, minced
- 2 cans (14 oz each) diced tomatoes
- 2 cups vegetable broth
- 1/4 cup fresh basil leaves, chopped
- Salt and pepper, to taste
- 1/4 cup plain Greek yogurt, for serving (optional)
- Fresh basil leaves, for garnish (optional)

Directions:
1. Heat olive oil in a large pot over medium heat. Add chopped onion and minced garlic, and cook until softened, about 5 minutes.
2. Add diced tomatoes (with their juices) and vegetable broth to the pot. Bring to a simmer and cook for 15 minutes.
3. Stir in chopped basil leaves and season with salt and pepper to taste.
4. Use an immersion blender to blend the soup until smooth. Alternatively, carefully transfer the soup to a blender and blend until smooth, then return to the pot.
5. Serve the tomato basil soup hot, with a dollop of plain Greek yogurt on top and garnished with fresh basil leaves if desired.

Nutritional Information (per serving):
- Calories: 100
- Protein: 3g

- Fat: 3g
- Carbohydrates: 16g
- Fiber: 5g

Coconut Curry Lentil Soup

Prep Time: 15 mins

Total Time: 45 mins

Servings: 4

Ingredients:

- 1 tablespoon olive oil
- 1 onion, chopped
- 2 cloves garlic, minced
- 2 carrots, diced
- 2 celery stalks, diced
- 1 cup dry red lentils, rinsed
- 4 cups vegetable broth
- 1 can (14 oz) coconut milk
- 2 tablespoons curry powder
- Salt and pepper, to taste
- Fresh cilantro, for garnish (optional)

Directions:

1. Heat olive oil in a large pot over medium heat. Add chopped onion and minced garlic, and cook until softened, about 5 minutes.
2. Add diced carrots and diced celery to the pot, and cook for another 5 minutes.

3. Stir in dry red lentils, vegetable broth, coconut milk, and curry powder. Bring to a simmer and cook for 25-30 minutes, or until lentils are tender.
4. Taste and adjust seasoning if necessary.
5. Serve the coconut curry lentil soup hot, garnished with fresh cilantro if desired.

Nutritional Information (per serving):
- Calories: 320
- Protein: 13g
- Fat: 18g
- Carbohydrates: 31g
- Fiber: 15g

SMOOTHIES RECIPES

Green Goddess Smoothie

Prep Time: 5 mins

Total Time: 5 mins

Servings: 2 glasses

Ingredients:

- 1 cup frozen organic blueberries
- 1/2 cup ice made with filtered or spring water
- 1 cup coconut water
- 1 1/2 cup greens (kale, spinach, or a mix)
- 1/2 avocado
- 1 tbsp. chia seeds
- 1 tsp honey (optional)
- Optional: a scoop of protein powder or collagen powder

Directions:

1. In a blender, combine the frozen blueberries, ice, coconut water, greens, avocado, chia seeds, and honey (if using).
2. Blend until smooth, adding more water if needed to reach your desired consistency.
3. Pour into glasses and enjoy immediately.

Nutritional Information (per serving):

- Calories: 220
- Protein: 5g
- Fat: 10g
- Carbohydrates: 30g

- Fiber: 10g

Berry Blast Smoothie

Prep Time: 5 mins

Total Time: 5 mins

Servings: 2 glasses

Ingredients:

- 1 cup frozen mixed berries (strawberries, raspberries, blueberries)
- 1/2 cup ice made with filtered or spring water
- 1 cup almond milk
- 1/2 ripe banana
- 1 tbsp. flaxseeds
- 1 tsp honey or maple syrup (optional)

Directions:

1. Combine the frozen mixed berries, ice, almond milk, ripe banana, flaxseeds, and honey or maple syrup (if using) in a blender.
2. Blend until smooth and creamy.
3. Pour into glasses and serve immediately.

Nutritional Information (per serving):

- Calories: 180
- Protein: 3g
- Fat: 5g
- Carbohydrates: 30g
- Fiber: 8g

Tropical Sunshine Smoothie

Prep Time: 5 mins

Total Time: 5 mins

Servings: 2 glasses

Ingredients:

- 1 cup frozen pineapple chunks
- 1/2 cup ice made with filtered or spring water
- 1 cup coconut water
- 1/2 ripe mango, peeled and diced
- 1/2 ripe banana
- 1/4 cup Greek yogurt
- Optional: a handful of spinach for extra greens

Directions:

1. Place the frozen pineapple chunks, ice, coconut water, ripe mango, banana, and Greek yogurt in a blender.
2. Blend until smooth and creamy.
3. Add spinach if desired and blend again until well combined.
4. Pour into glasses and serve immediately.

Nutritional Information (per serving):

- Calories: 200
- Protein: 5g
- Fat: 2g
- Carbohydrates: 40g
- Fiber: 6g

Chocolate Peanut Butter Protein Smoothie

Prep Time: 5 mins

Total Time: 5 mins

Servings: 2 glasses

Ingredients:

- 2 ripe bananas
- 1 cup almond milk
- 2 tbsp. peanut butter
- 2 tbsp. cocoa powder
- 1 scoop chocolate protein powder
- 1/2 cup ice made with filtered or spring water
- Optional: a drizzle of honey or maple syrup for sweetness

Directions:

1. Add ripe bananas, almond milk, peanut butter, cocoa powder, protein powder, and ice to a blender.
2. Blend until smooth and creamy.
3. If desired, add honey or maple syrup for additional sweetness and blend again.
4. Pour into glasses and enjoy immediately.

Nutritional Information (per serving):

- Calories: 280
- Protein: 18g
- Fat: 10g
- Carbohydrates: 35g
- Fiber: 7g

Detox Green Smoothie

Prep Time: 5 mins

Total Time: 5 mins

Servings: 2 glasses

Ingredients:

- 1 cup spinach
- 1/2 cup kale
- 1/2 cucumber, peeled and chopped
- 1 green apple, cored and chopped
- 1/2 lemon, juiced
- 1 cup coconut water
- 1/2 cup ice made with filtered or spring water
- Optional: a knob of ginger for added flavor

Directions:

1. Combine spinach, kale, cucumber, green apple, lemon juice, coconut water, ice, and ginger (if using) in a blender.
2. Blend until smooth and creamy.
3. Pour into glasses and serve immediately.

Nutritional Information (per serving):

- Calories: 100
- Protein: 3g
- Fat: 1g
- Carbohydrates: 25g
- Fiber: 7g

Berry Protein Smoothie

Prep Time: 5 mins

Total Time: 5 mins

Servings: 2 glasses

Ingredients:

- 1 cup frozen mixed berries (strawberries, blueberries, raspberries)
- 1/2 cup almond milk
- 1/2 cup Greek yogurt
- 1 scoop vanilla protein powder
- 1 tbsp chia seeds
- 1/2 banana
- 1/2 cup ice made with filtered or spring water

Directions:
1. Combine frozen mixed berries, almond milk, Greek yogurt, protein powder, chia seeds, banana, and ice in a blender.
2. Blend until smooth and creamy.
3. If the smoothie is too thick, add more water to achieve the desired consistency.
4. Pour into glasses and serve immediately.

Nutritional Information (per serving):
- Calories: 250
- Protein: 25g
- Fat: 6g
- Carbohydrates: 25g
- Fiber: 8g

Pineapple Coconut Smoothie

Prep Time: 5 mins
Total Time: 5 mins
Servings: 2 glasses

Ingredients:

- 1 cup frozen pineapple chunks
- 1/2 cup coconut milk
- 1/2 cup Greek yogurt
- 1/2 banana
- 1 tbsp shredded coconut
- 1/2 cup ice made with filtered or spring water

Directions:

1. In a blender, combine frozen pineapple chunks, coconut milk, Greek yogurt, banana, shredded coconut, and ice.
2. Blend until smooth and creamy.
3. Add more water if needed for desired consistency.
4. Pour into glasses and serve immediately.

Nutritional Information (per serving):

- Calories: 220
- Protein: 7g
- Fat: 10g
- Carbohydrates: 30g
- Fiber: 6g

Mango Avocado Smoothie

Prep Time: 5 mins

Total Time: 5 mins

Servings: 2 glasses

Ingredients:

- 1 cup frozen mango chunks
- 1/2 avocado
- 1/2 cup almond milk

- 1/2 cup Greek yogurt
- 1 tbsp honey
- 1/2 cup ice made with filtered or spring water

Directions:
1. In a blender, combine frozen mango chunks, avocado, almond milk, Greek yogurt, honey, and ice.
2. Blend until smooth and creamy.
3. Adjust consistency with more water if necessary.
4. Pour into glasses and serve immediately.

Nutritional Information (per serving):
- Calories: 240
- Protein: 8g
- Fat: 8g
- Carbohydrates: 35g
- Fiber: 6g

Green Tea Smoothie

Prep Time: 5 mins
Total Time: 5 mins
Servings: 2 glasses

Ingredients:
- 1 cup brewed green tea, cooled
- 1/2 cup frozen pineapple chunks
- 1/2 cup spinach
- 1/2 banana
- 1/2 cup Greek yogurt
- 1 tbsp honey

- 1/2 cup ice made with filtered or spring water

Directions:
1. Brew green tea and let it cool.
2. In a blender, combine cooled green tea, frozen pineapple chunks, spinach, banana, Greek yogurt, honey, and ice.
3. Blend until smooth and creamy.
4. Adjust consistency with more water if needed.
5. Pour into glasses and serve immediately.

Nutritional Information (per serving):
- Calories: 210
- Protein: 7g
- Fat: 2g
- Carbohydrates: 40g
- Fiber: 5g

Chocolate Banana Peanut Butter Smoothie

Prep Time: 5 mins

Total Time: 5 mins

Servings: 2 glasses

Ingredients:
- 1 cup almond milk
- 1 banana
- 2 tbsp cocoa powder
- 2 tbsp peanut butter
- 1 scoop chocolate protein powder
- 1/2 cup ice made with filtered or spring water

Directions:

1. In a blender, combine almond milk, banana, cocoa powder, peanut butter, protein powder, and ice.
2. Blend until smooth and creamy.
3. Adjust consistency with more water if necessary.
4. Pour into glasses and serve immediately.

Nutritional Information (per serving):
- Calories: 280
- Protein: 18g
- Fat: 10g
- Carbohydrates: 30g
- Fiber: 8g

Green Detox Smoothie

Prep Time: 5 mins
Total Time: 5 mins
Servings: 2 glasses

Ingredients:
- 1 cup spinach
- 1/2 cucumber, peeled and chopped
- 1/2 green apple, cored and chopped
- 1/2 avocado
- 1/2 lemon, juiced
- 1/2 cup coconut water
- 1/2 cup ice made with filtered or spring water
- Optional: 1 tsp honey or sweetener of choice

Directions:

1. Combine spinach, cucumber, green apple, avocado, lemon juice, coconut water, and ice in a blender.
2. Blend until smooth and creamy.
3. Taste and add honey or sweetener if desired.
4. Pour into glasses and serve immediately.

Nutritional Information (per serving):

- Calories: 120
- Protein: 3g
- Fat: 7g
- Carbohydrates: 14g
- Fiber: 6g

Berry Blast Smoothie

Prep Time: 5 mins

Total Time: 5 mins

Servings: 2 glasses

Ingredients:

- 1 cup mixed berries (strawberries, blueberries, raspberries)
- 1/2 banana
- 1/2 cup Greek yogurt
- 1/2 cup almond milk
- 1 tbsp chia seeds
- 1/2 cup ice made with filtered or spring water

Directions:

1. Place mixed berries, banana, Greek yogurt, almond milk, chia seeds, and ice in a blender.
2. Blend until smooth.

3. Add more water if needed to reach desired consistency.
4. Pour into glasses and serve immediately.

Nutritional Information (per serving):
- Calories: 160
- Protein: 7g
- Fat: 4g
- Carbohydrates: 24g
- Fiber: 8g

Tropical Paradise Smoothie

Prep Time: 5 mins

Total Time: 5 mins

Servings: 2 glasses

Ingredients:
- 1/2 cup pineapple chunks
- 1/2 cup mango chunks
- 1/2 banana
- 1/2 cup coconut milk
- 1/2 cup ice made with filtered or spring water
- Optional: 1 tbsp shredded coconut

Directions:
1. Combine pineapple chunks, mango chunks, banana, coconut milk, and ice in a blender.
2. Blend until smooth.
3. Add shredded coconut if desired and blend briefly.
4. Pour into glasses and serve immediately.

Nutritional Information (per serving):

- Calories: 180
- Protein: 2g
- Fat: 8g
- Carbohydrates: 30g
- Fiber: 5g

Creamy Peanut Butter Smoothie

- **Prep Time:** 5 mins
- **Total Time:** 5 mins
- **Servings:** 2 glasses

Ingredients:

- 2 tbsp natural peanut butter
- 1 banana
- 1 cup spinach
- 1/2 cup Greek yogurt
- 1/2 cup almond milk
- 1/2 cup ice made with filtered or spring water

Directions:

1. In a blender, combine peanut butter, banana, spinach, Greek yogurt, almond milk, and ice.
2. Blend until smooth.
3. Adjust thickness with more water if needed.
4. Pour into glasses and serve immediately.

Nutritional Information (per serving):

- Calories: 240
- Protein: 10g
- Fat: 14g

- Carbohydrates: 21g
- Fiber: 5g

Chia Berry Smoothie Bowl

Prep Time: 5 mins

Total Time: 5 mins

Servings: 2 bowls

Ingredients:

- 1 cup mixed berries (strawberries, blueberries, raspberries)
- 1/2 banana
- 1/2 cup Greek yogurt
- 2 tbsp chia seeds
- 1/2 cup almond milk
- Toppings: sliced banana, granola, shredded coconut (optional)

Directions:

1. Blend mixed berries, banana, Greek yogurt, chia seeds, and almond milk until smooth.
2. Pour into bowls.
3. Top with sliced banana, granola, and shredded coconut if desired.
4. Serve immediately.

Nutritional Information (per serving):

- Calories: 180
- Protein: 8g
- Fat: 5g
- Carbohydrates: 25g
- Fiber: 9g

Protein-Packed Berry Blast Smoothie

Prep Time: 5 mins

Total Time: 5 mins

Servings: 2 glasses

Ingredients:

- 1 cup mixed berries (strawberries, blueberries, raspberries)
- 1/2 banana
- 1/2 cup Greek yogurt
- 1 scoop protein powder (whey or plant-based)
- 1/2 cup almond milk
- 1 tbsp chia seeds
- 1/2 cup ice made with filtered or spring water

Directions:

1. Combine mixed berries, banana, Greek yogurt, protein powder, almond milk, chia seeds, and ice in a blender.
2. Blend until smooth and creamy.
3. Adjust consistency by adding more water if needed.
4. Pour into glasses and serve immediately.

Nutritional Information (per serving):

- Calories: 250
- Protein: 20g
- Fat: 7g
- Carbohydrates: 30g
- Fiber: 8g

Green Power Smoothie

Prep Time: 5 mins

Total Time: 5 mins

Servings: 2 glasses

Ingredients:

- 2 cups spinach
- 1/2 cucumber, peeled and chopped
- 1/2 avocado
- 1/2 cup coconut water
- 1/2 cup pineapple chunks
- 1/2 lime, juiced
- 1/2 cup ice made with filtered or spring water

Directions:

1. Blend spinach, cucumber, avocado, coconut water, pineapple chunks, lime juice, and ice until smooth.
2. Adjust consistency with additional water if necessary.
3. Pour into glasses and serve immediately.

Nutritional Information (per serving):

- Calories: 180
- Protein: 4g
- Fat: 10g
- Carbohydrates: 22g
- Fiber: 8g

Creamy Peanut Butter Banana Smoothie

Prep Time: 5 mins

Total Time: 5 mins

Servings: 2 glasses

Ingredients:

- 2 tbsp natural peanut butter
- 1 banana
- 1/2 cup Greek yogurt
- 1/2 cup almond milk
- 1/2 cup ice made with filtered or spring water

Directions:

1. In a blender, combine peanut butter, banana, Greek yogurt, almond milk, and ice.
2. Blend until smooth and creamy.
3. Add more water if needed to reach desired consistency.
4. Pour into glasses and serve immediately.

Nutritional Information (per serving):

- Calories: 280
- Protein: 14g
- Fat: 15g
- Carbohydrates: 25g
- Fiber: 5g

Turmeric Mango Smoothie

Prep Time: 5 mins

Total Time: 5 mins

Servings: 2 glasses

Ingredients:

- 1 cup frozen mango chunks
- 1/2 banana
- 1/2 cup Greek yogurt
- 1/2 tsp ground turmeric

- 1/2 tsp ground ginger
- 1/2 cup almond milk
- 1/2 cup ice made with filtered or spring water

Directions:
1. Blend mango chunks, banana, Greek yogurt, turmeric, ginger, almond milk, and ice until smooth.
2. Adjust thickness with additional water if desired.
3. Pour into glasses and serve immediately.

Nutritional Information (per serving):
- Calories: 160
- Protein: 7g
- Fat: 3g
- Carbohydrates: 28g
- Fiber: 4g

Antioxidant Superfood Smoothie

Prep Time: 5 mins

Total Time: 5 mins

Servings: 2 glasses

Ingredients:
- 1 cup mixed berries (strawberries, blueberries, raspberries)
- 1/2 cup spinach
- 1/2 cup kale
- 1/2 cup Greek yogurt
- 1/2 cup almond milk
- 1 tbsp honey
- 1/2 cup ice made with filtered or spring water

Directions:
1. Blend mixed berries, spinach, kale, Greek yogurt, almond milk, honey, and ice until smooth.
2. Adjust sweetness with more honey if desired.
3. Pour into glasses and serve immediately.

Nutritional Information (per serving):
- Calories: 180
- Protein: 8g
- Fat: 3g
- Carbohydrates: 30g
- Fiber: 7g

MEAL PLAN

Day 1
- **Breakfast:** Protein-Packed Berry Blast Smoothie
- **Lunch:** Grilled Chicken Salad
- **Dinner:** Baked Salmon with Steamed Vegetables

Day 2
- **Breakfast:** Green Power Smoothie
- **Lunch:** Quinoa Salad with Chickpeas and Avocado
- **Dinner:** Turkey Meatballs with Zucchini Noodles

Day 3
- **Breakfast:** Creamy Peanut Butter Banana Smoothie
- **Lunch:** Lentil Soup with Whole Grain Bread
- **Dinner:** Grilled Shrimp with Brown Rice and Roasted Vegetables

Day 4
- **Breakfast:** Turmeric Mango Smoothie
- **Lunch:** Greek Yogurt Parfait with Berries and Granola
- **Dinner:** Baked Chicken Breast with Sweet Potato Mash and Green Beans

Day 5
- **Breakfast:** Antioxidant Superfood Smoothie
- **Lunch:** Spinach and Feta Omelette with Whole Wheat Toast
- **Dinner:** Vegetable Stir-Fry with Tofu and Quinoa

Day 6

- **Breakfast:** Protein-Packed Berry Blast Smoothie
- **Lunch:** Mediterranean Chickpea Salad
- **Dinner:** Grilled Fish Tacos with Cabbage Slaw

Day 7

- **Breakfast:** Green Power Smoothie
- **Lunch:** Caprese Salad with Whole Grain Bread
- **Dinner:** Butternut Squash Soup with Grilled Chicken Salad

Day 8

- **Breakfast:** Creamy Peanut Butter Banana Smoothie
- **Lunch:** Lentil Salad with Roasted Vegetables
- **Dinner:** Baked Salmon with Quinoa and Steamed Broccoli

Day 9

- **Breakfast:** Turmeric Mango Smoothie
- **Lunch:** Greek Yogurt Parfait with Almonds and Honey
- **Dinner:** Turkey Chili with Mixed Greens Salad

Day 10

- **Breakfast:** Antioxidant Superfood Smoothie
- **Lunch:** Vegetable Soup with Whole Grain Crackers
- **Dinner:** Stir-Fried Tofu with Brown Rice and Vegetables

Day 11

- **Breakfast:** Protein-Packed Berry Blast Smoothie
- **Lunch:** Quinoa Salad with Roasted Chickpeas and Avocado

- **Dinner:** Grilled Chicken Breast with Sweet Potato Mash and Green Beans

Day 12
- **Breakfast:** Green Power Smoothie
- **Lunch:** Greek Salad with Grilled Shrimp
- **Dinner:** Vegetable Curry with Basmati Rice

Day 13
- **Breakfast:** Creamy Peanut Butter Banana Smoothie
- **Lunch:** Caprese Sandwich with Mixed Greens Salad
- **Dinner:** Baked Cod with Roasted Vegetables

Day 14
- **Breakfast:** Turmeric Mango Smoothie
- **Lunch:** Chickpea and Spinach Stew with Whole Grain Bread
- **Dinner:** Grilled Vegetable Skewers with Quinoa Pilaf

Day 15
- **Breakfast:** Antioxidant Superfood Smoothie
- **Lunch:** Lentil Soup with Whole Wheat Pita
- **Dinner:** Baked Chicken Thighs with Cauliflower Rice and Steamed Broccoli

Day 16
- **Breakfast:** Protein-Packed Berry Blast Smoothie
- **Lunch:** Greek Yogurt Parfait with Walnuts and Berries
- **Dinner:** Turkey Meatballs with Marinara Sauce and Zucchini Noodles

Day 17

- **Breakfast:** Green Power Smoothie
- **Lunch:** Quinoa Salad with Roasted Vegetables and Feta Cheese
- **Dinner:** Grilled Salmon with Asparagus and Brown Rice

Day 18

- **Breakfast:** Creamy Peanut Butter Banana Smoothie
- **Lunch:** Mixed Greens Salad with Grilled Chicken and Balsamic Vinaigrette
- **Dinner:** Vegetable Stir-Fry with Tofu and Brown Rice

Day 19

- **Breakfast:** Turmeric Mango Smoothie
- **Lunch:** Greek Salad with Grilled Shrimp
- **Dinner:** Lentil and Vegetable Curry with Basmati Rice

Day 20

- **Breakfast:** Antioxidant Superfood Smoothie
- **Lunch:** Caprese Sandwich with Mixed Greens Salad
- **Dinner:** Baked Cod with Quinoa Pilaf and Steamed Broccoli

Day 21

- **Breakfast:** Protein-Packed Berry Blast Smoothie
- **Lunch:** Lentil Soup with Whole Grain Bread
- **Dinner:** Grilled Chicken Breast with Roasted Vegetables

CONCLUSION

In conclusion, the journey through various dietary recipes tailored for individuals with EPI (Exocrine Pancreatic Insufficiency) has been both enlightening and enriching. EPI presents unique challenges in nutrient absorption, requiring careful consideration of ingredients and cooking methods to optimize digestion and overall health. Throughout this exploration, we have delved into a plethora of recipes spanning smoothies, soups, seafood dishes, desserts, and snacks, each meticulously crafted to provide nourishment while accommodating the dietary needs of those with EPI.

Smoothies emerged as versatile options, blending nutrient-dense fruits, vegetables, and healthy fats to create delicious and easily digestible beverages. With ingredients like organic blueberries, coconut water, greens, and avocado, these smoothies offer a refreshing way to boost nutrient intake and support gut health. By incorporating optional additions such as turmeric and protein powder, these recipes can be customized to address specific health concerns and dietary preferences.

Soups proved to be another valuable addition to the EPI diet, offering warmth, comfort, and ample nutrition in each spoonful. From hearty lentil soups to creamy butternut squash blends, these recipes showcase the versatility of ingredients like legumes, vegetables, and lean proteins in creating satisfying meals. Coupled with whole grain bread or crackers, soups provide a balanced combination of carbohydrates, protein, and fiber, promoting satiety and stable blood sugar levels.

Seafood dishes provided an abundance of omega-3 fatty acids and lean protein, essential for supporting heart health and muscle function.

Whether it's grilled salmon, baked cod, or shrimp tacos, these recipes offer delicious ways to incorporate seafood into the EPI diet. Paired with nutrient-rich sides like quinoa, brown rice, or steamed vegetables, seafood dishes contribute to a well-rounded and satisfying meal plan.

Desserts, while typically associated with indulgence, were reimagined to align with the EPI diet's nutritional goals. By utilizing wholesome ingredients like fruits, nuts, and natural sweeteners, desserts became nourishing treats rather than empty calories. From fruit salads to chia seed puddings, these recipes demonstrate that satisfying cravings can be achieved without compromising health.

Snacks rounded out the meal plan, providing convenient options for refueling between meals. With choices ranging from microbiome smoothies to nutrient-packed trail mix, these snacks offer a balance of macronutrients and micronutrients to support energy levels and curb hunger throughout the day.

In navigating the complexities of EPI, one thing remains clear: prioritizing health is paramount. As Hippocrates famously said, "Let food be thy medicine and medicine be thy food." By embracing nutrient-dense ingredients, mindful cooking practices, and a holistic approach to nutrition, individuals with EPI can optimize their well-being and enhance their quality of life. Each recipe presented here serves as a testament to the transformative power of food in promoting health and vitality. As we continue on our journey towards wellness, let us remember that every bite we take is an opportunity to nourish our bodies and nurture our souls.

In closing, may these recipes serve as a source of inspiration and empowerment on your path to better health. Remember that small changes can yield significant results, and every step taken towards prioritizing self-care is a step towards a brighter, healthier future. Let us embrace the journey with gratitude, curiosity, and resilience, knowing that we have the power to shape our health and wellness through the choices we make each day.

www.ingramcontent.com/pod-product-compliance
Lightning Source LLC
Chambersburg PA
CBHW052159220526
45471CB00004B/1742